SCLEROTHERAPY OF SPIDER VEINS

It is worthwhile to secure the happiness of the patient as well as to prolong his life.
WILLIAM J. MAYO (1861–1939)

SCLEROTHERAPY OF SPIDER VEINS

VICTORIA VITALE-LEWIS, M.D., F.A.C.S.

Medical Illustrator
ANNE SISSON, M.F.A., A.M.I.

BUTTERWORTH-HEINEMANN

Boston   Oxford   Melbourne   Singapore   Toronto   Munich   New Delhi   Tokyo

Copyright © 1995 by Butterworth-Heinemann

℞ A member of the Reed Elsevier group

All rights reserved.

Every effort has been made to ensure that the drug dosage schedules within this text are accurate and conform to standards accepted at time of publication. However, as treatment recommendations vary in the light of continuing research and clinical experience, the reader is advised to verify drug dosage schedules herein with information found on product information sheets. This is especially true in cases of new or infrequently used drugs.

♾ Recognizing the importance of preserving what has been written, Butterworth-Heinemann prints its books on acid-free paper whenever possible.

Library of Congress Cataloging-in-Publication Data
Vitale-Lewis, Victoria.
    Sclerotherapy of spider veins / Victoria Vitale-Lewis ; medical
illustrator, Anne Sisson.
        p. cm.
    Includes bibliographical references and index.
    ISBN 0-7506-9459-9 (alk. paper)
    1. Varicose veins—Treatment. 2. Varicose veins—Treatment—
Atlases. 3. Solutions, Sclerosing. I. Sisson, Anne. II. Title.
    [DNLM: 1. Telangiectasis—therapy—atlases. 2. Sclerotherapy—
methods—atlases. WG 17 V836s 1995]
    RC695.V55 1995
    616.1'4306—dc20
    DNLM/DLC
    for Library of Congress   95–14198
                                                                CIP

British Library Cataloguing-in-Publication Data
A catalogue record for this book is available from the British Library.

Butterworth-Heinemann
313 Washington Street
Newton, MA 02158-1626

10 9 8 7 6 5 4 3 2 1

Printed in the United States of America

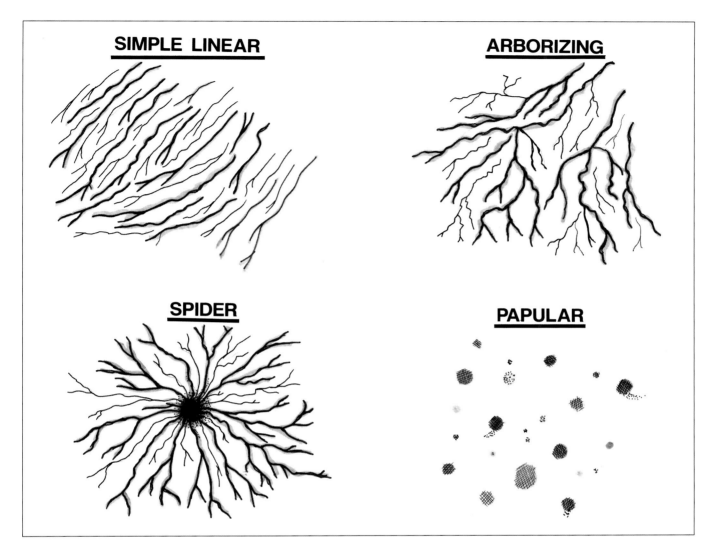

SIMPLE LINEAR

ARBORIZING

SPIDER

PAPULAR

FIGURE 1–1. *Four patterns of telangiectasias. A. Simple linear. B. Arborizing. C. Spider. D. Papular. (From Redisch W, Pelzer RH: Am Heart J 1949; 37: 106.)*

PATTERNS OF SPIDER VEINS

Spider veins can occur anywhere on the lower extremities. They commonly occur in certain patterns in particular locations. These patterns are similar to those described by Redisch in other areas of the body[4] (Fig. 1–1). The arborizing types are definitely easier to sclerose than the simple types, since fewer punctures are necessary to sclerose a significant number of vessels when they are connected in a arborizing fashion. On the lateral thigh, the spider veins commonly resemble a cartwheel, where arborizing groups of spider veins radiate around a

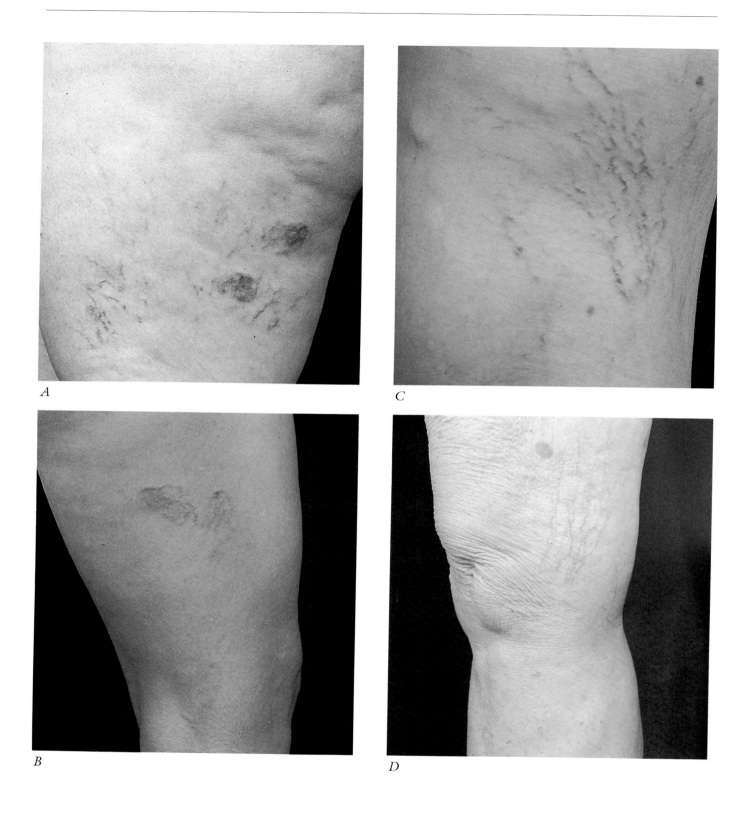

A

B

C

D

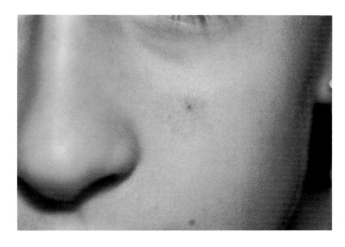

FIGURE 1–3. *Spider telangiectasia of the cheek. Note central arteriole with radiating limbs.*

central point, as shown in Figure 1–2A. At times, a reticular vein is seen as this central point leading into the spider veins (Fig. 1–2B,C). On the medial knee area, the spider veins usually occur in a more longitudinal fashion[5] (Fig. 1–2D).

MORPHOLOGY OF SPIDER VEINS

Spider veins of the lower extremities differ from telangiectasias in other areas of the body in morphology as well as physiology. The spider telangiectasia usually found on the face, hands, and arms but rarely below the umbilicus is formed by a central arteriole[6] (Fig. 1–3). Biopsies of spider veins on the lower extremities have confirmed their identify as small veins rather than arteries.[7] Since they are actually small veins, they are subject in a dampened fashion to the ambulatory venous pressure that is developed in the standing position. These differences between spider veins of the lower extremities and telangiectasias elsewhere on the body may account for the differences in effectiveness of various treatment modalities that have been applied to each.

FIGURE 1–2. *A. Arborizing "cartwheel" pattern of telangiectasias common on lateral thigh. B,C. Reticular vein on each thigh leading directly into spider veins. D. Linear pattern of telangiectasias common on medial knee.*

REFERENCES

1. Engel A, Johnson ML, Haynes SG. Health effects of sunlight exposure in the United States: Results from the first national health and nutrition examination survey, 1971–1974. Arch Dermatol 1988; 124:72–79.

2. Weiss RA, Weiss MA. Resolution of pain associated with varicose and telangiectatic leg veins after compression sclerotherapy. J Dermatol Surg Oncol 1990; 16:333–336.

3. Weiss MA, Weiss RA, Goldman MP. How minor varicosities cause leg pain. Contemp Obstet Gynecol 1991; 36:113–125.

4. Redisch W, Pelzer RH. Localized vascular dilatations of the human skin: Capillary microscopy and related studies. Am Heart J 1949;37:106–112.

5. Green AR, Morgan BDG. Sclerotherapy for venous flare. Br J Plast Surg 1985; 38:241–242.

6. Olsen T. Peripheral vascular diseases and vascular-related diseases. In Moschella SL, Hurley HJ, eds: Dermatology, 2d ed. Vol 2. Philadelphia: WB Saunders, 1985, pp 1000–1086.

7. Bodian EL. Techniques of sclerotherapy for sunburst venous blemishes. J Dermatol Surg Oncol 1985; 11:696–704.

ADDITIONAL READINGS

Biegeleisen K. Primary lower extremity telangiectasias: relationship of size to color. Angiology 1987; 38:760–768.

de Faria JL, Moraes IN. Histopathology of the telangiectasia associated with varicose veins. Dermatologic 1963; 127:321–329.

Ouvry PA, Davy A. The sclerotherapy of telangiectasia. Phlébologie 1982; 35: 349–359.

Wokalek H, Vanscheidt W, Martay K et al. Morphology and localization of sunburst varicosities: An electron microscopic and morphometric study. J Dermatol Surg Oncol 1989;15:149–154.

2

ANATOMY AND PATHOPHYSIOLOGY OF THE VENOUS SYSTEM

CERTAINLY THE MAJORITY of patients presenting with spider veins have no clinical evidence of varicose veins or deep venous disease. However, there are some patients with spider veins in certain locations that may be the only clinical presentation of underlying venous disease, most notably in the ankle area. Knowledge of the basic anatomy and physiology of the venous system is necessary to adequately evaluate patients who present only with the complaint of unsightly spider veins before initiating sclerotherapy.

The venous system of the lower extremities consists of the superficial venous system and the deep venous system, and they are connected by the perforating veins. The superficial veins are located for the most part superficial to the muscle fascia, while the deep veins are below the fascia. During relaxation of the muscles, the deep venous system fills with deoxygenated blood from the superficial system via the one-way-valved perforating veins. Contraction of the calf muscles during exercise such as walking propels this blood back to the heart. Reflux of blood back to the superficial system is prevented by the one-way valves of the perforating veins, which are squeezed closed during contraction. Reflux of blood distally is also prevented by closed one-way valves distally (Fig. 2–1A,B).

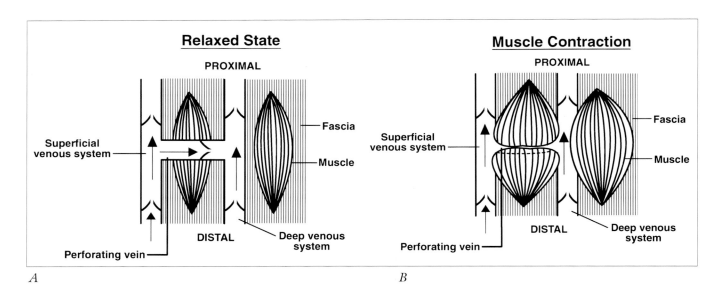

F I G U R E 2–1. *A. During muscle relaxation, the one-way valves of the perforating veins allow blood flow from the superficial to the deep venous system. B. During muscle contraction, the blood is propelled proximally. The closed one-way valves prevent reflux both distally and into the superficial system.*

S U P E R F I C I A L V E N O U S S Y S T E M

The superficial venous system consists primarily of the long and short saphenous veins and their tributaries. The long saphenous vein is first visible at approximately ankle level anterior to the medial malleolus, originating from the medial end of the dorsal venous arch. It courses up the anteromedial aspect of the leg, posterior to the medial aspect of the knee, and then along the anteromedial aspect of the thigh to empty into the deep venous system in the groin at the saphenofemoral junction (Fig. 2–2). The short saphenous vein is first seen on the lateral ankle posterior to the lateral malleolus and then travels up the posterior leg to empty into the deep venous system just above the posterior knee at the saphenopopliteal junction (Fig. 2–3). Valves are also present along these conduit vessels to prevent reflux distally in the standing position. Reflux in the superficial system results in the development of primary varicosities.

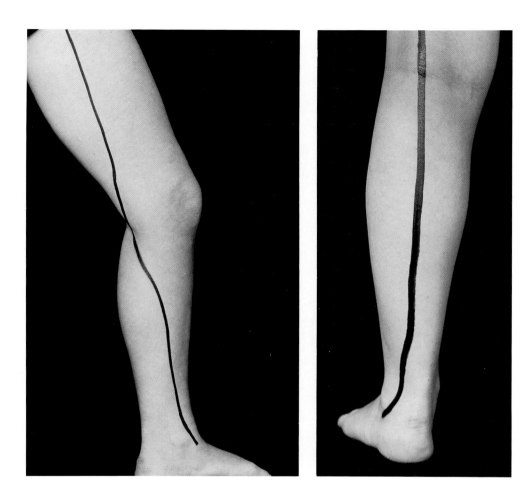

FIGURE 2–2. *The path of the long saphenous vein anterior to the medial malleolus, up the medial aspect of the leg, posterior to the medial knee, and along the anteromedial aspect of the thigh to the saphenofemoral junction in the groin.*

FIGURE 2–3. *The path of the short saphenous vein from the posterior to the lateral malleolus, up the posterior leg to the saphenopopliteal junction just above the posterior knee.*

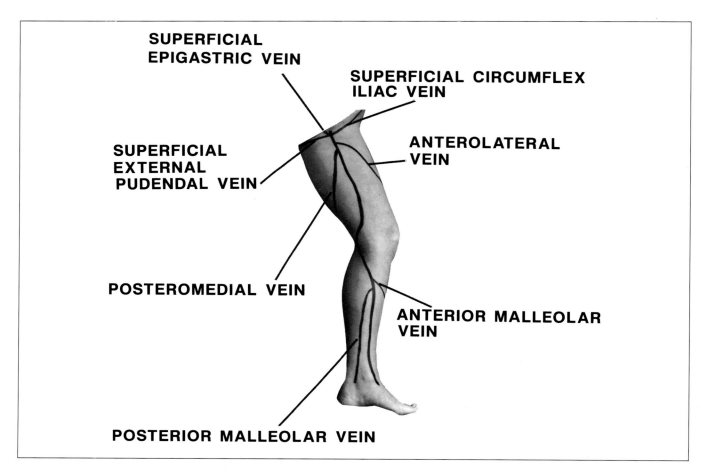

SUPERFICIAL EPIGASTRIC VEIN

SUPERFICIAL CIRCUMFLEX ILIAC VEIN

SUPERFICIAL EXTERNAL PUDENDAL VEIN

ANTEROLATERAL VEIN

POSTEROMEDIAL VEIN

ANTERIOR MALLEOLAR VEIN

POSTERIOR MALLEOLAR VEIN

FIGURE 2–4.
Tributaries of the long saphenous vein.

The long saphenous vein is accompanied in the leg by a branch of the saphenous nerve and in the thigh by the anterior femoral cutaneous nerve. Important tributaries of the long saphenous vein include the anterior and posterior malleolar veins in the leg, the anterolateral and posteromedial veins in the thigh, and the superficial circumflex iliac, the superficial epigastric, and the superficial external pudendal veins at the saphenofemoral junction (Fig. 2–4 and Table 2–1). The most important tributary in the lower leg is the posterior malleolar vein, which is also popularly known as the "vein of Leonard." It is located just posterior to the long saphenous vein and receives the Cockett perforators in the leg from the deep venous system.

TABLE 2–1. *Tributaries of Long Saphenous Vein*
Long Saphenous Vein
Tributaries in Leg
Ant. Malleolar Vein
Post Malleolar Vein (Vein of Leonard)
Tributaries in Thigh
Anterolateral Vein
Posteromedial Vein
Tributaries at Saphenofemoral Junction
Superficial Circumflex Iliac Vein
Superficial Epigastric Vein
Superficial External Pudendal Vein

Important tributaries of the long saphenous system in the thigh include the anterolateral vein, formally called the *accessary saphenous vein*, and the posteromedial vein. The anterolateral vein originates laterally on the lower thigh and courses superomedially to join the long saphenous vein distal to the saphenofemoral junction. The posteromedial vein begins on the lower posterior thigh and courses around the medial aspect of the middle thigh to empty into the long saphenous vein distal to the saphenofemoral junction.

Three tributaries enter the long saphenous vein at its junction with the femoral vein. Paralleling the groin crease from the upper lateral to the medial thigh is the superficial circumflex iliac vein. The superficial inferior epigastric vein extends obliquely downward on the anterior abdominal wall to the saphenofemoral junction. The superficial external pudendal vein courses transversely along the upper medial thigh just below the perineal crease. Each of these veins accompanies an artery of the same name.

Incompetency of the saphenofemoral junction can lead to primary varicosities of the long saphenous vein and any of its tributaries. It is important to note that the external pudendal veins are also connected to the ovarian veins via the pelvic veins. Reflux from this pelvic source can give rise to varicosities in the medial thigh through the external pudendal veins.

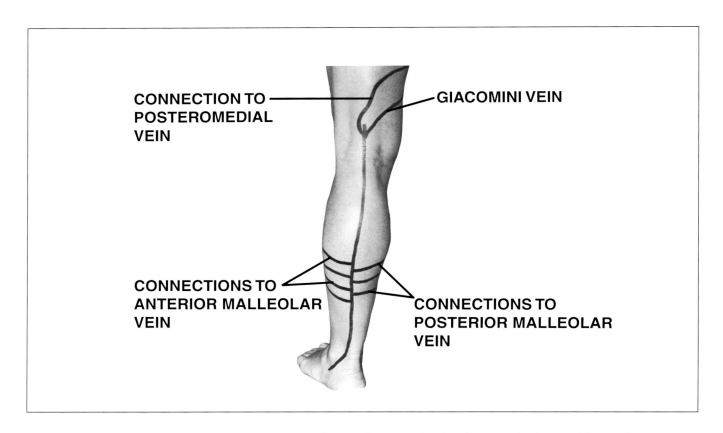

FIGURE 2–5. *Usual communications between the short and long saphenous veins. These communicating veins can transmit reflux in the long saphenous vein to the short saphenous vein.*

The short saphenous vein originates on the lateral aspect of the foot and travels posterior to the lateral malleolus and then superiorly up to the posterior aspect of the leg to pierce the crural fascia between the heads of the gastrocnemius muscle at about the midleg level. It continues superiorly to terminate usually in the popliteal vein at the saphenopopliteal junction just above the level of the knee fold. It is accompanied in the ankle and lower to middle leg by the sural nerve. Important tributaries of the short saphenous vein are those which communicate with the long saphenous vein, because they can transmit incompetency in the long saphenous system to the short saphenous system (Fig. 2–5). The most significant is the Giacomini vein, which arises from the short saphenous vein at its subaponeurotic level and courses around the medial aspect of the thigh to empty into the long saphenous vein.

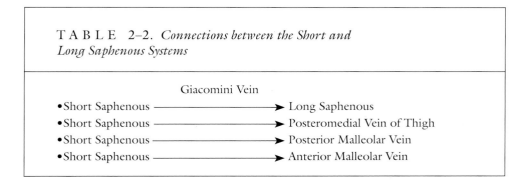

TABLE 2–2. *Connections between the Short and Long Saphenous Systems*
Giacomini Vein
• Short Saphenous ⟶ Long Saphenous
• Short Saphenous ⟶ Posteromedial Vein of Thigh
• Short Saphenous ⟶ Posterior Malleolar Vein
• Short Saphenous ⟶ Anterior Malleolar Vein

Three other routes connect the long and short saphenous systems. Tributaries of the short saphenous connect with the posteromedial vein of the lower posterior thigh, with the posterior malleolar vein around the medial aspect of the leg, and with the anterior malleolar vein around the lateral aspect of the leg (Table 2–2).

DEEP VENOUS SYSTEM

A working knowledge of the anatomy of the deep venous system is essential to properly evaluate a patient who presents with only the complaint of spider veins in order to rule out any underlying venous disease. There are two components to the deep venous system, the conducting veins and the sinusoidal veins.[1]

The conducting veins represent the outflow tract for the blood back to the heart; the sinusoidal veins are located   the muscles and serve as reservoirs to collect the blood that is propelled back to the heart on muscle contraction through the conducting system.

The conducting deep veins accompany the arteries of the same names in the subfascial compartments. The deep veins of the leg are paired and include the anterior tibial veins in the anterior compartment, the posterior tibial veins in the posterior compartment, and the peroneal veins in the lateral compartment. The posterior tibial and peroneal veins unite to form the tibioperoneal trunk. These veins are then joined by the anterior tibial veins to form the popliteal vein at a variable level in the

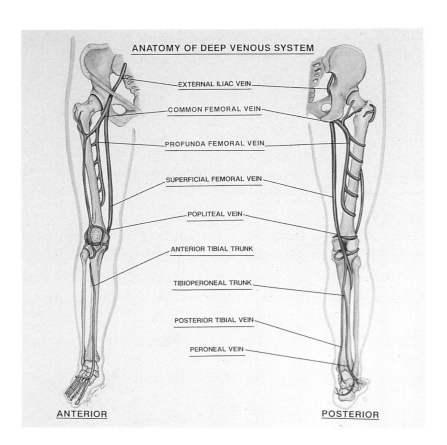

FIGURE 2–6. *The usual anatomy of the deep venous system of the lower extremity.*

popliteal fossa. The popliteal vein then travels superiorly behind the knee, is joined by the short saphenous vein at the sapheno-popliteal junction, and finally becomes the superficial femoral vein at the adductor hiatus in the lower thigh. In the thigh, the superficial femoral vein is joined by the profunda femoral vein to form the common femoral vein at a variable distance below the inguinal ligament. At the fossa ovalis just below the inguinal ligament, the long saphenous vein empties into the common femoral vein. Passing under the inguinal ligament, the common femoral vein becomes the external iliac vein (Fig. 2–6). The sinusoidal deep veins are located in the calf within the gastrocnemius and soleus muscles. These venous sinuses are filled with blood during muscle relaxation and empty through the conducting veins on muscle contraction.

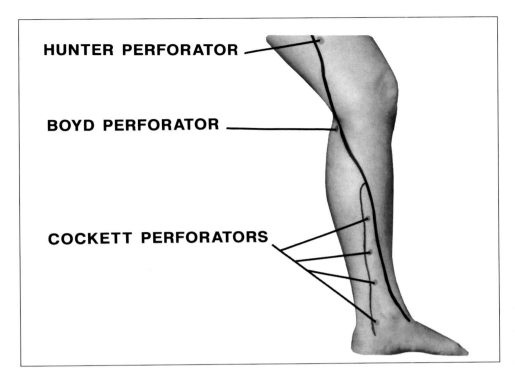

FIGURE 2-7. *The most common locations of perforating veins associated with the long saphenous system.*

In the image:

HUNTER PERFORATOR

BOYD PERFORATOR

COCKETT PERFORATORS

PERFORATING VEINS

The perforating veins join the superficial and deep systems. They contain valves which allow the blood to flow from the superficial to the deep systems, and prevent reflux back into the superficial system. Some have direct paths between the superficial and deep systems, whereas others have indirect paths communicating with the muscular venous channels before emptying into the deep system. The perforating veins are many in number. Several studies have been performed to localize the most constant perforators, which can be the sites of reflux from the deep to the superficial system in the pathologic state.

There are five constant perforators from the long saphenous vein or its tributaries to the deep venous system (Fig. 2–7). In the middle to lower thigh, approximately 15 cm above the knee, the Hunter perforator connects the long saphenous vein with the superficial femoral vein at Hunter's canal. In the leg just below the knee and just behind the

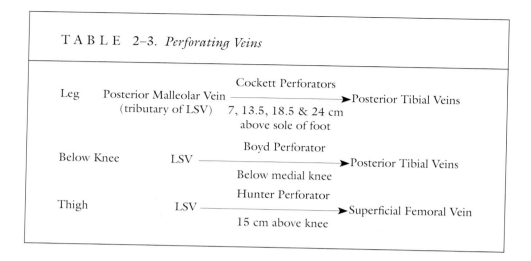

TABLE 2–3. *Perforating Veins*

Leg	Posterior Malleolar Vein (tributary of LSV)	Cockett Perforators ⟶ 7, 13.5, 18.5 & 24 cm above sole of foot	Posterior Tibial Veins
Below Knee	LSV	Boyd Perforator ⟶ Below medial knee	Posterior Tibial Veins
Thigh	LSV	Hunter Perforator ⟶ 15 cm above knee	Superficial Femoral Vein

tibia, the Boyd perforator connects the long saphenous system with the posterior tibial veins. In the middle to lower leg, there are three Cockett perforators that connect the posterior arch vein, a tributary of the long saphenous vein, to the posterior tibial veins. The most superior is located on the posteromedial aspect of the leg just posterior to the tibia and approximately 18 cm above the sole of the foot. The middle and lower Cockett perforators are also located along Linton's line (vertical line one finger breadth posterior to the medial malleolus) 7.0 and 13.5 cm above the sole of the foot. Just above the Cockett perforators, there is a fourth perforating vein lying along the same vertical line 24.0 cm above the foot[2] (Table 2–3).

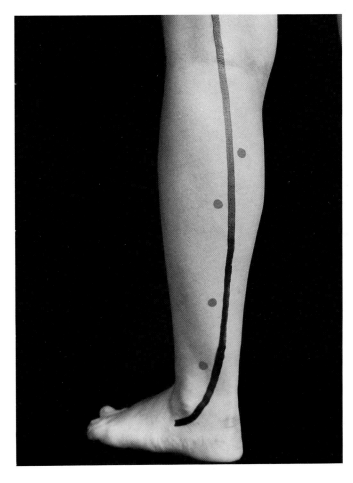

FIGURE 2–8. *The most common locations of the perforating veins associated with the short saphenous system.*

The most constant perforators related to the short saphenous vein are located on the posterolateral aspect of the leg. Most of these perforators join the lateral arch vein, a tributary of the short saphenous vein to the peroneal vein (Fig. 2–8).

REFERENCES

1. Tibbs DJ. Varicose Veins and Related Disorders. Oxford: Butterworth-Heinemann, 1992, 5–10.
2. May R. Nomenclature of the surgically most important connecting veins. In May R, Partsch H, Straubesand J, eds. Perforating Veins. Munich: Urban & Schwarzenberg, 1981, 13–18.

ADDITIONAL READINGS

Beesley WH, Fegan WG. An investigation into the localization of incompetent perforating veins. Br J Surg 1970; 57: 30–32.

Bracey, DW. Simple device for location of perforating veins. Br Med J 1958; 2: 101–102.

Dodd H, Cockett FB. The Pathology and Surgery of the Veins of the Lower Limbs, 2d ed. New York: Churchill-Livingstone, 1976.

Lawrence D, Fish PJ, Kakkar VV. Blood-flow in incompetent perforating veins. Lancet 1977; 1: 117–118.

Linton RR. The communicating veins of the lower leg and the operative technic for their ligation. Ann Surg 1938; 107: 582–593.

McMullin GM, Scott HJ, Smith PDC, Scurr JH. A reassessment of the role of perforating veins in chronic venous insufficiency. Phlebology 1990; 5:85–94.

Miller SS, Foote AV. The ultrasonic detection of incompetent perforating veins. Br J Surg 1974; 61:653–656.

Noble J, Gunn AA. Varicose veins: Comparative study of methods for detecting incompetent perforators. Lancet 1972; 1:1253–1255.

O'Donnell TF, Burnand KG, Clemenson G, et al. Doppler examination vs clinical and phlebographic detection of the location of incompetent perforating veins. Arch Surg 1977; 112:31–35.

Papadakis K, Christodoulou C, Christopoulos D, et al. Number and anatomical distribution of incompetent thigh perforating veins. Br J Surg 1989; 76:581–584.

Sherman RS. Varicose veins: Anatomic findings and an operative procedure based upon them. Ann Surg 1944; 772–784.

Stolic E. Terminology, division, and systematic anatomy of the communicating veins of the lower limb. In May R, Partsch H, Straubesand J, eds: Perforating Veins. Munich: Urban & Schwarzenberg, 1981, pp 19–34.

Strandness DE Jr, Thiele BL. Selected Topics in Venous Disorders: Pathophysiology, Diagnosis, and Treatment. New York: Futura, 1981.

Thomson H. The surgical anatomy of the superficial and perforating veins of the lower limb. Ann R Coll Surg Engl 1979; 61:198–205.

Woodburne RT. Essentials of Human Anatomy, 5th ed. New York: Oxford University Press, 1973.

Zukowski AJ, Nicolaides AN, Szendro G, et al. Haemodynamic significance of incompetent calf perforating veins. Br J Surg 1991; 78:625–629.

3

PATIENT SELECTION AND EXAMINATION

PROPER PATIENT SELECTION is essential to the success of sclerotherapy of spider veins. The physician must first ascertain if the patient is a suitable candidate for the procedure. A thorough history and physical examination with emphasis on pertinent factors relating to the venous system are the key to proper patient selection.

HISTORY

The first fact to establish is that the patient's venous disease is limited to spider veins (Table 3–1). At times the patient can point out areas of bulging varicosities that appear only after prolonged standing and certainly require evaluation. Any symptoms related to the spider veins by the patient must be noted. Usually the patient's primary concern is the appearance of the spider veins. Previous treatment of veins is certainly important information, including previous surgeries or sclerotherapy and the success of that treatment. It is imperative to question the patient about any past history of deep vein thrombosis, superficial thrombophlebitis, pulmonary embolism, and leg ulcers to ascertain those patients who may warrant an extensive venous evaluation. Previous leg injuries should be reviewed for any relevant information relating to altered anatomy especially of the venous system.

Name of Patient _____ Age _____

Name of Husband, Wife, or Friend to call in case of Emergency _____

When did you first notice your spider viens? _____

Have the veins in your legs ever been treated? _____

  If yes, by surgery? _____ When? _____

  By injections? _____ When? _____

  What was injected? _____

Which leg is worse? _____

Right _____ Left _____ Same _____

Have you ever had surgery? _____

  What kind? _____

  When/Where? _____

Have you had any serious illness, accidents, or previous
  hospitalizations? _____

List _____

_____

_____

Are you allergic to any medications? _____

List _____

_____

_____

What medications are you presently taking? _____

_____

_____

Are you taking any of the following medications?

____ Aspirin   ____ Water Pills

____ Pain Pills   ____ Tranquilizers

____ Blood Pressure Pills   ____ Antihistamines

____ Birth Control Pills   ____ Estrogen

____ Recreational Drugs

Do you have any of the following habits?

____ Smoking   Freq. _____ Amt. _____

____ Drinking   Freq. _____ Amt. _____

Have you suffered from?

____ Fainting   ____ Dizziness

____ Heart Disease   ____ Heart Murmurs

____ Rheumatic Fever   ____ Chest Pain

____ High Blood Pressure   ____ Asthma

____ Yellow jaundice   ____ Hepatitis

____ Easy Bruising   ____ Diabetes

____ Thyroid Disease   ____ Arthritis

____ Blood clots in legs   ____ Phlebitis

____ Leg Ulcers   ____ Leg Injury

____ Pain or cramping in legs

____ Blood clots in Lungs (Pulmonary embolus)

Have you ever been told you have "poor circulation?" ____

Are you pregnant? _____

Last menstrual period _____

Have you been trying or is a chance you might be
  pregnant? _____

How many times have you been pregnant? _____

Did your spider veins worsen after pregnancy? _____

Are you currently breast feeding? _____

Do any of your family members suffer from varicose
or spider veins? _____

Please List: _____

_____

Do your veins:

____ Ache   ____ Swell   ____ Itch

____ Become Red   ____ Become Tender

Does the appearance of your spider veins bother you?

_____

Do you have or have you had any communicable
  diseases? _____

Is there any chance you could have AIDS or have you ever
  had contact with an AIDS victim? _____

Have you had blood tranfusions? _____

Have you ever used intravenous street drugs? _____

Height _____

Weight _____

Name of General Physician _____

_____

Name of Gynecologist _____

_____

Second, the physician should inquire about predisposing factors to the development of these spider veins, such as pregnancy, topical steroid use, or hormonal therapy. A positive family history of varicose veins or spider veins usually can be elicited. Information obtained about daily activities, such as the patient's job and exercise routine, may uncover some lifestyle adaptations that could be made to prevent further stress on the venous system of the lower extremities, such as avoidance of prolonged sitting or standing.

Third, the history must include direct questioning about any contraindications or relative contraindications to sclerotherapy. These include questions regarding current medical conditions such as pregnancy or nursing. History of allergies to medications or asthma may influence the choice of the sclerosant to be used. Past history of deep vein thrombosis, superficial thrombophlebitis, or leg ulcers serves as a warning sign of underlying venous disease that must be properly evaluated. Any symptom of arterial insufficiency of the lower extremities also must be evaluated by physical examination and perhaps by other testing. Ischemia and diabetic neuropathy pose additional risks of nonhealing if ulceration should result as a complication of sclerotherapy. Sclerotherapy should not be performed while the patient is suffering from a febrile illness or a blood-borne disease such as hepatitis or acquired immunodeficiency syndrome (AIDS). The age of a patient is only a consideration; mobility rather than advanced age is the key issue. Episodes of deep vein thrombosis have been reported in cases of sclerotherapy of spider veins only. The patient must be able to walk following the procedure in order to try to avoid this serious complication.

PHYSICAL EXAMINATION

Examine the entire extent of the lower extremities in the standing position. The superficial venous system cannot be examined adequately in the supine position because gravity is the precipitating factor of the venous ambulatory pressure. An organized approach to examination of the lower extremities that is followed in every patient ensures accuracy and thoroughness.

There are three basic steps to the examination of every patient presenting for sclerotherapy of spider veins:

1. Inspection
2. Mapping
3. Palpation

Inspection

First, the patient's legs must be inspected from above the groin to the feet bilaterally and circumferentially with the patient in the standing position. Allow the patient to stand in one place for a few minutes before examining in order to promote venous distension. The room should not be cold to avoid venoconstriction.

The locations of all the spider veins from the groin to the toes circumferentially are inspected. The patient is often quite aware of the exact locations of all the spider veins that are of concern to him or her. Be careful to inspect all these areas, including the ones the patient points out in particular. The patient may be bothered by spider veins that may be too small to be sclerosed. One must be very honest with the patient concerning the suitability of the problematic spider veins for sclerotherapy and the realistic results that can be achieved. Also, the physician must mentally note the number of spider veins the patient is interested in ablating in order to plan the appropriate time necessary for the treatment plan to be accomplished. It is also useful to note the most involved extremity and/or area so that there is a basis of comparison as the treatment plan progresses without constantly referring to the preoperative photographs. In other words, the patient may wish to start the sclerotherapy in the most involved area so that the improvement can be compared with lesser involved areas to check the progress of the sclerotherapy. Also, it is imperative to note any reticular veins that may be feeding the spider veins, because these also must be sclerosed in order for the sclerotherapy of the spider veins to be successful in the long term. Attention then should be turned to examination of the major tributary territories of the superficial venous system, as discussed in the section on anatomy. The paths of the long and short saphenous veins and their important tributaries should be inspected in order to avoid missing any major reflux in the superficial venous system. If there are any bulging varicosities, certainly these must be noted.

The limb also must be inspected for any signs of chronic venous insufficiency such as edema, fibrosis, venostasis, dermatitis, or evidence of old leg ulcers. The sites of any scars or evidence of previous trauma to the lower extremity must be noted for two reasons. The physician certainly does not want to be held accountable for scars that were present prior to sclerotherapy. Also, the scars may indicate previous surgery or injury to the venous system that the patient may have not divulged in the history. The patient's pigmentation should be documented prior to proceeding with the sclerotherapy. Especially in the older patients and smokers, examination of the foot for coolness, blanching on elevation, or rubor on dependency should alert the physician to possible peripheral vascular disease.

Mapping

As the physician inspects the legs, it is often convenient at the same time to make a map of the spider veins as well as the reticular veins and any other findings of significance on inspection. These maps are very useful as the treatment progresses in serving as a very rapid reference to the presclerotherapy extent of the spider veins. The large drawings indicated in Figure 3–1 are useful in the permanent record, and make it quite easy to map the veins rapidly.

Palpation

It is very helpful to run your hands down the legs of any patient who has a significant number of spider veins so as to detect any bulging varicosities that may have been missed visually. The fingers are sometimes more sensitive than the eye in picking up the bulging character of any significantly dilated veins.

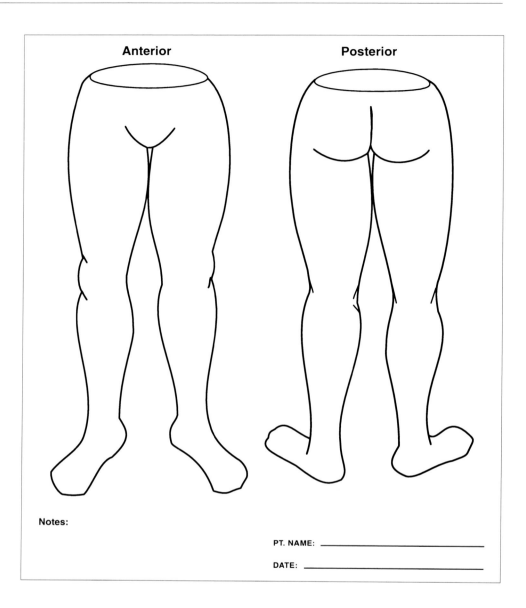

Anterior   Posterior

Notes:

PT. NAME: _____

DATE: _____

FIGURE 3–1.
Convenient template for
mapping of spider veins.

There were some palpation tests described years ago that can be useful in certain patients. These tests are useful only if bulging veins are seen or palpated.

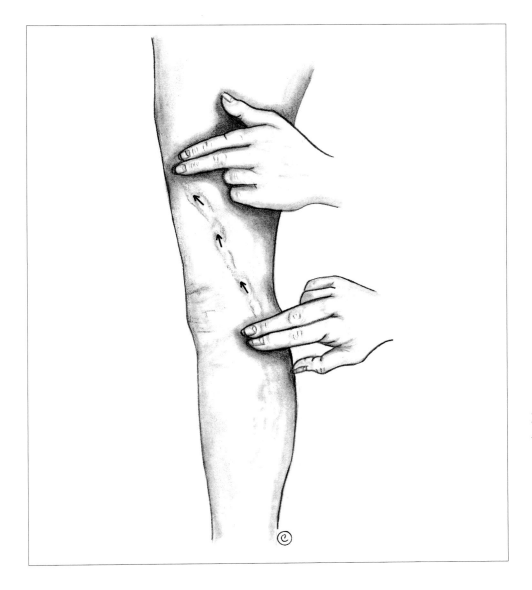

FIGURE 3–2.
A palpable thrill produced by tapping over the course of the vein indicates an abnormally large volume of blood being displaced by the tap, suggestive of significant reflux. This can be useful for mapping the course of the reflux to the highest point.

SCHWARTZ TEST (FIG. 3–2). This involves tapping over the path of a dilated vein with the opposite hand placed over the vein path either above or below the tapping finger. If a thrill is felt with the opposite hand, then an abnormally large volume of blood is being displaced by the tap, suggestive of significant reflux. This test can be helpful in tracing the path of a varicosity to either the long or short saphenous system.

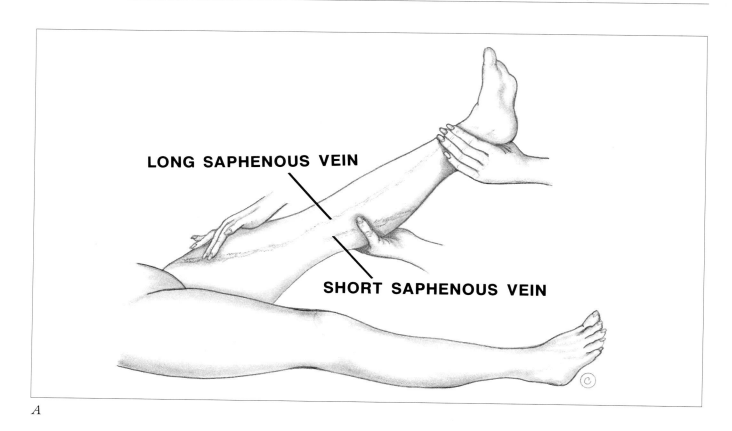

LONG SAPHENOUS VEIN

SHORT SAPHENOUS VEIN

A

FIGURE 3–3. *Trendelenburg test for reflux in the short and/or long saphenous veins. A. Leg is elevated and emptied of blood. B. With finger pressure over proximal long and short saphenous veins, the patient stands. C. The finger is released first from the short saphenous vein. Venous bulging indicates reflux. D. The finger is then released from the long saphenous vein. E. Bulging of the long saphenous vein indicates reflux. Concomitant development of dilatation of the short saphenous vein indicates transmission of reflux from the long to the short saphenous vein.*

TRENDELENBURG TEST (FIG. 3–3). The leg is emptied of blood, and a finger is placed over both the proximal long and the short saphenous veins. The patient stands, and the fingers are released from the short saphenous vein and then from the long saphenous vein. Rapid filling of the vein upon release of the finger pressure proximally indicates incompetency of the short or long saphenous veins. This test also can be used to tell if the short saphenous vein is actually incompetent or rather is filling from the long saphenous vein.

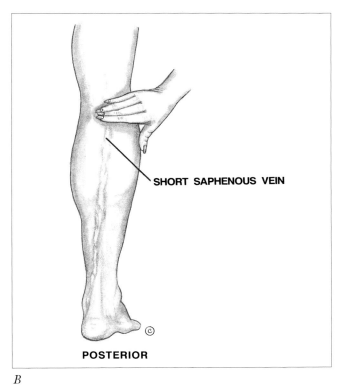

SHORT SAPHENOUS VEIN

POSTERIOR

B

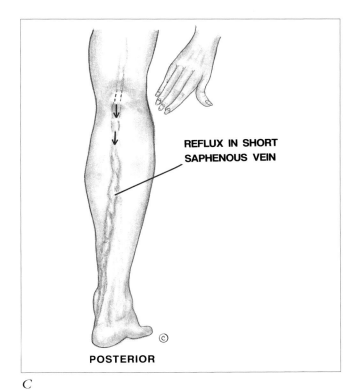

REFLUX IN SHORT
SAPHENOUS VEIN

POSTERIOR

C

LONG SAPHENOUS VEIN

ANTERIOR

D

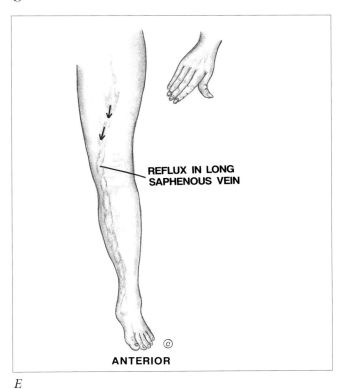

REFLUX IN LONG
SAPHENOUS VEIN

ANTERIOR

E

FIGURE 3–3. (Continued)

Patient Selection and Examination

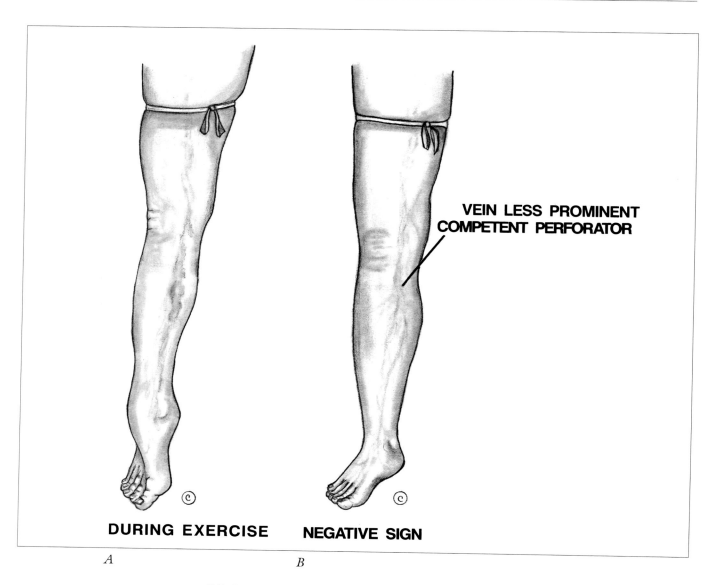

DURING EXERCISE **NEGATIVE SIGN**

VEIN LESS PROMINENT COMPETENT PERFORATOR

A   *B*

FIGURE 3–4. *Perthes test for incompetency of a perforating vein. A. Patient rises up on toes to exercise calf muscles. Tourniquet is placed to block the superficial venous system, and patient exercises again. B. Negative test. If clinically the superficial veins become less distended, the perforator is competent. C. Negative test. Physiologically, the blood is draining from the superficial to the deep system and then proximally, with backflow prohibited by competent valves.*

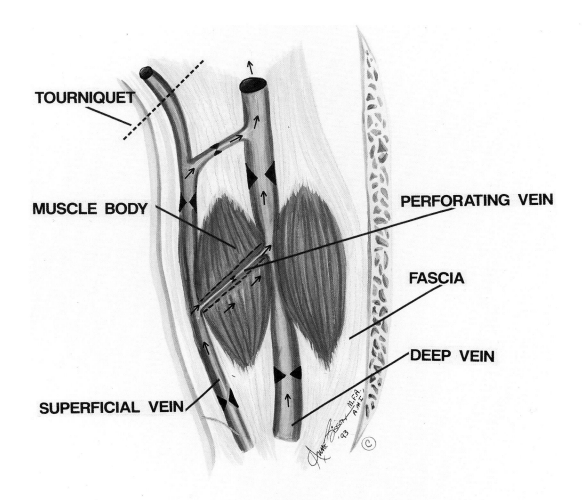

TOURNIQUET

MUSCLE BODY

PERFORATING VEIN

FASCIA

DEEP VEIN

SUPERFICIAL VEIN

C　　　**NEGATIVE SIGN**

C

PERTHES TEST (FIG. 3–4). This test was designed to demonstrate incompetency of a perforating vein. The patient exercises the calf muscles by rising on his or her toes several times. A tourniquet is applied proximally to block the superficial venous system. Then the calf muscles are exercised again. If the superficial veins become less distended, the perforator is felt to be competent, with normal draining from the superficial to the deep venous system with exercise. If the veins become more distended, the perforator is felt to be incompetent, with the blood refluxing from the deep to the superficial system on exercise.[1]

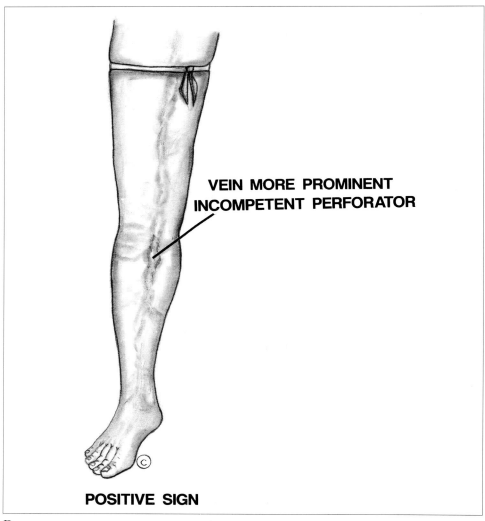

**VEIN MORE PROMINENT
INCOMPETENT PERFORATOR**

POSITIVE SIGN

D

FIGURE 3–4. (Continued)
D. Positive test. If clinically the superficial veins become more distended, the perforator is incompetent. E. Positive test. Physiologically, the blood is refluxing from the deep to the superficial system through the incompetent valves of the perforating vein.

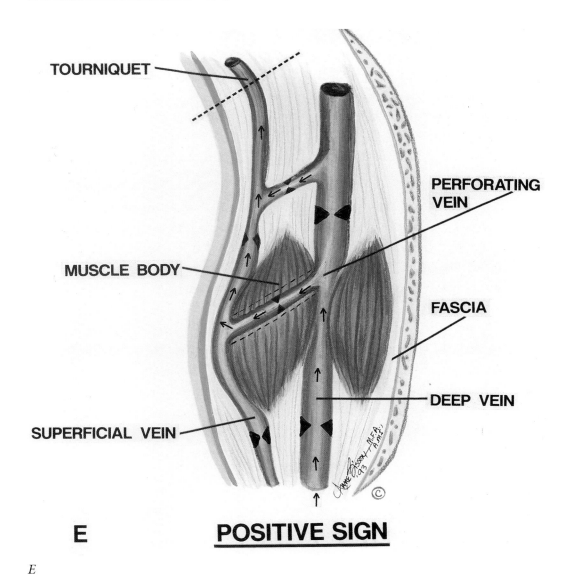

POSITIVE SIGN

E

E

F I G U R E 3–4. *Continued*

Obviously, these palpation tests are useful only in the cases of dilated veins. There are three primary objectives to the careful clinical examination of the lower extremities in every patient who presents with a complaint of cosmetically unacceptable spider veins:

1. The practitioner must rule out the presence of bulging varicosities. Thorough inspection and palpation of the paths of the long and short saphenous veins and their major tributaries and the sites of common perforators, as well as all the areas in which the spider veins are present, ensures that no bulging varicosities were missed clinically.

2. The practitioner must rule out any signs of chronic venous insufficiency or arterial insufficiency.

3. The practitioner must accurately map the location of all the spider veins, reticular veins, old scars, or pigment changes. Once the practitioner has documented the presence of only minor telangiectatic "spider veins," then no other further testing is required, and the telangiectasias may be treated with sclerotherapy.[2]

The presence of any reticular veins, bulging varicosities, or chronic venous insufficiency requires further noninvasive testing of the venous system, as discussed in the next chapter. These additional diagnostic techniques should be considered only if warranted by abnormal clinical findings on a thorough history and physical examination. The performance of these tests on cosmetic patients with minor telangiectasias is an unnecessary expense to the health care system.

REFERENCES

1. Dodd H, Cockett FB. The Pathology and Surgery of the Veins of the Lower Limb. London: Churchill-Livingstone, 1976, pp 84–85.
2. Goldman MP, Fronek A. Anatomy and pathophysiology of varicose veins. J Dermatol Surg Oncol 1989; 15:138–145.

ADDITIONAL READINGS

Alexander CJ. Chair-sitting and varicose veins. Lancet 1972; 1:822–823.

Beaglehole R. Epidemiology of varicose veins. World J Surg 1986; 10:898–902.

Brand FN, Dannenberg AL, Abbott RD, Kannel WB. The epidemiology of varicose veins: The Framingham Study. Am J Prevent Med 1988; 4:96–101.

Dodd H. The cause, prevention, and arrest of varicose veins. Lancet 1964; 2:809–811.

Gundersen J, Hauge M. Hereditary factors in venous insufficiency. Angiology 1969; 20:346–355.

McEnroe CS, O'Donnell TF, Mackey WC. Correlation of clinical findings with venous hemodynamics in 386 patients with chronic venous insufficiency. Am J Surg 1988; 156:148–152.

O'Donnell TF Jr., McEnroe CS, Heggerick P. Chronic venous insufficiency. Surg Clin North Am 1990; 70:159–166.

Rose SS, Ahmed A. Some thoughts on the aetiology of varicose veins. J Cardiovasc Surg 1986; 27:534–543.

Sadick NS. Predisposing factors of varicose and telangiectatic leg veins. J Dermatol Surg Oncol 1992; 18:883–886.

Sadick NS, Niedt GW. A study of estrogen and progesterone receptors in spider telangiectasias of the lower extremities. J Dermatol Surg Oncol 1990; 16:620–623.

Tibbs DJ. Recognizing the abnormal: Clinical examination and the special tests. In Tibbs DJ, ed: Varicose Veins and Related Disorders. Oxford: Butterworth-Heinemann, 1992, pp 30–42.

Vin F, Allaert FA, Levardon M. Influence of estrogens and progesterone on the venous system of the lower limbs in women. J Dermatol Surg Oncol 1992; 18:888–892.

Noninvasive Testing of the Venous System

THERE ARE MANY METHODS of noninvasive testing of the venous system. Many of these methods require the purchase of expensive machinery to determine if obstruction or reflux of the venous system is present, to establish the volume of the reflux, and to visualize the sites of reflux and obstruction. These expensive methods of venous testing are necessary to adequately evaluate the venous system if the patient has significant venous disease such as chronic venous insufficiency or dilated varicosities on clinical examination. However, most of these expensive machines are impractical and unnecessary purchases for the practitioner interested in the sclerotherapy of spider veins only.

Many patients who present with spider veins also will have some reticular veins of questionable significance as far as the volume of reflux present. For example, only 22.9 percent of patients with spider veins were found to have superficial venous incompetence in a study by Thibault that evaluated cosmetic-like veins.[1] The incompetency was largely in the long saphenous system from below the knee upward. These patients may be treated by sclerotherapy but may require stronger sclerosing agents in greater concentrations and may benefit by postsclerotherapy compression. If the practitioner is unsure if significant reflux is present after examining the patient clinically, then Doppler ultrasound may be helpful.

35

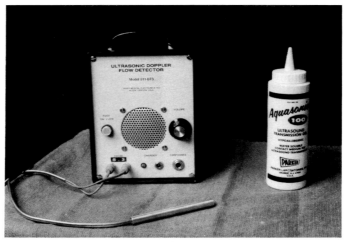

A

FIGURE 4–1. *A. One model of a Doppler ultrasound and acoustic gel. B. The Doppler ultrasound emits an ultrasound beam of a particular frequency from the transmitting crystal. A frequency shift (Doppler effect) is caused by moving red blood cells, and the backscattered ultrasound beam is picked up by the receiving crystal.*

DOPPLER ULTRASOUND

The hand-held Doppler ultrasound device is an inexpensive, portable, and easy method to examine the venous system noninvasively. The reliability of the results depends on the practitioner's expertise in conducting the examination. However, with a little practice, the practitioner can rapidly become quite adept in examination of the venous system using the Doppler ultrasound.

The Doppler ultrasound can be as small as pocket-size and has a probe that contains a pizeoelectric crystal (Fig. 4–1). The device contains an oscillator that vibrates at a certain frequency. A frequency of 8 MHz is optimal for examination of the venous system. The oscillator causes the pizeoelectric crystal to admit an ultrasound beam. Acoustic gel is placed on the skin to allow transmission of the beam. A frequency shift (Doppler effect) is caused by moving red blood cells in the path of the beam which is received by a second crystal in the probe. This output can be projected audibly or as a waveform. The probe is held at a 45–degree angle with the skin for optimal transmission.

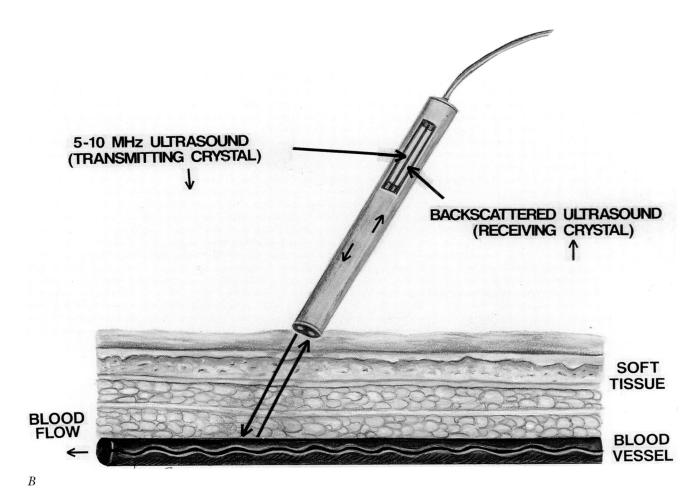

5-10 MHz ULTRASOUND (TRANSMITTING CRYSTAL)

BACKSCATTERED ULTRASOUND (RECEIVING CRYSTAL)

SOFT TISSUE

BLOOD FLOW

BLOOD VESSEL

B

F I G U R E 4–1. *(Continued)*

Certain maneuvers of examination give valuable information about the competency and patency of the venous system. There are three basic "normal" responses to ultrasound maneuvers (Table 4–1). These responses are better elicited with the patient in the standing position.

T A B L E 4–1. *Normal Responses to Ultrasound Maneuvers*

Distal Compression: Augmentation
Proximal Compression: Obliteration
Release of Proximal Compression: Augmentation

---

1. Compression distal to the probe normally should cause movement of blood through an unobstructed venous system proximally, augmenting the venous signal.

2. Compression proximal to the probe should result in obliteration of the venous flow and hence the Doppler output.

3. When the proximal compression is released, there should be an increased venous outflow again, creating an augmented signal. (Fig. 4–2).

FIGURE 4–2. *Normal responses to ultrasound maneuvers. A,B. Compression distal to the probe forces blood proximally, augmenting the Doppler signal. C,D. Compression proximal to the probe obliterates the venous flow and the Doppler signal. E,F. Release of proximal compression results in increased venous outflow, augmenting the Doppler signal.*

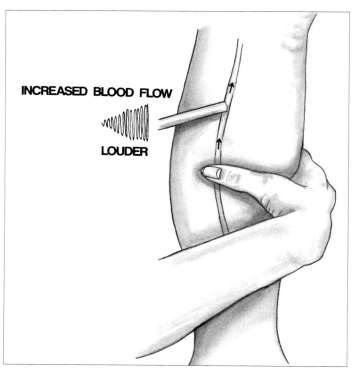

INCREASED BLOOD FLOW

LOUDER

A

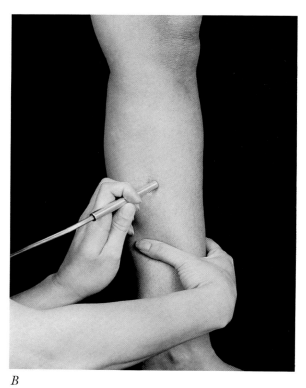

B

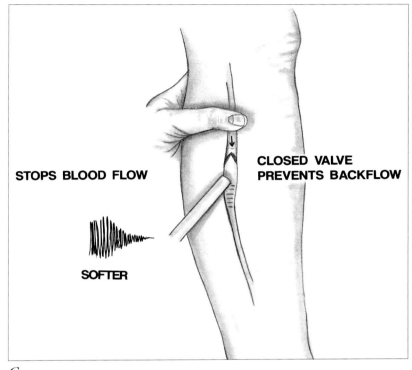

STOPS BLOOD FLOW

CLOSED VALVE PREVENTS BACKFLOW

SOFTER

C

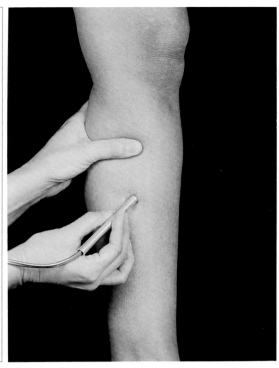

D

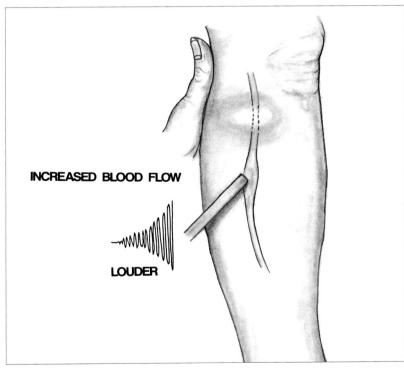

INCREASED BLOOD FLOW

LOUDER

E

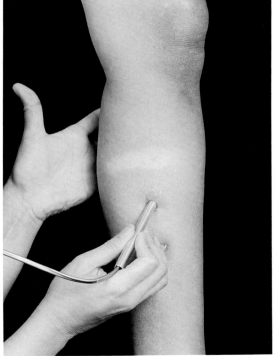

F

T A B L E   4–2. *Reflux: Responses to Ultrasound Maneuvers*

Proximal Compression: Augmentation
Release of Distal Compression: Augmentation

The abnormal responses to maneuvers that are pathognomonic of reflux in the examined vein are augmentation produced by proximal compression and augmentation on release of distal compression (Table 4–2). Distal compression normally pushes the blood proximally, creating an augmented signal. When the distal compression is released, the augmentation of the signal should cease unless reflux is present in the vein. In this case, the additional blood propelled upward by the distal compression now refluxes downward through incompetent valves, creating augmentation of the Doppler signal on release of distal compression. Compression proximal to the probe normally should obliterate the venous outflow and hence the Doppler signal. If there is reflux in the vein, proximal compression will propel the venous blood downward through incompetent valves, producing an abnormal augmentation of the venous system by proximal compression (Fig. 4–3).

Venous obstruction decreases venous outflow, resulting in a dampened ultrasound signal. The abnormal responses to the maneuvers that are pathognomonic of venous obstruction depend on probe placement in relation to the site of obstruction. If the obstruction is distal to the

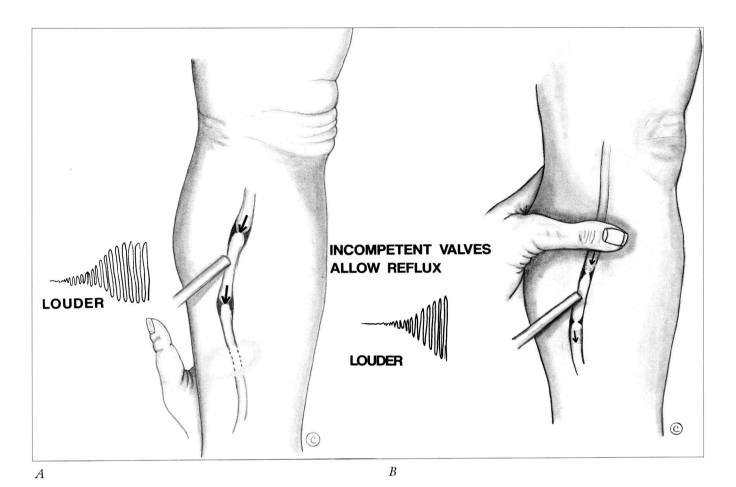

LOUDER

INCOMPETENT VALVES
ALLOW REFLUX

LOUDER

A

B

F I G U R E 4–3. *Reflux: Responses to Ultrasound maneuvers. A. On release of distal compression, the enlarged volume of blood refluxes back downward through the incompetent valves, augmenting the Doppler signal. B. Compression proximal to probe increases reflux downward through the incompetent valves, augmenting the Doppler signal.*

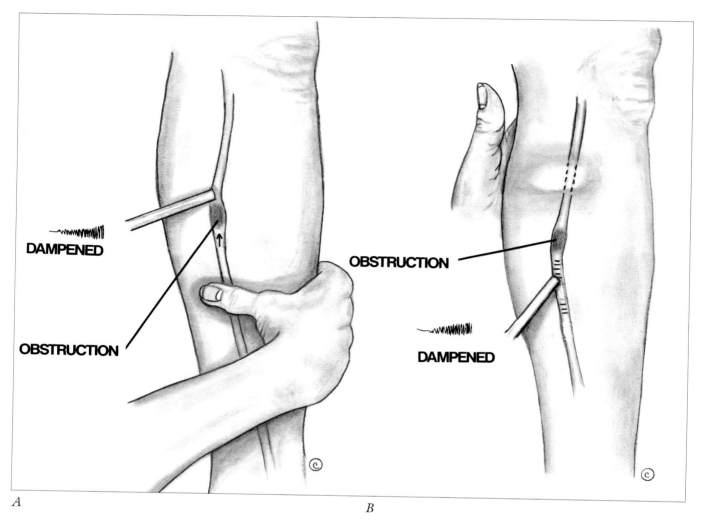

DAMPENED

OBSTRUCTION

OBSTRUCTION

DAMPENED

A

B

FIGURE 4-4. *Venous obstruction: Responses to Ultrasound maneuvers. A. Obstruction distal to the Doppler probe blocks the increased blood flow usually created by distal compression, resulting in dampening of the usual augmentation. B. Obstruction proximal to the Doppler probe blocks the increased blood flow usually created by release of proximal compression, resulting in dampening of the usual augmentation.*

probe, then one can expect a dampening of the usual augmentation created by the distal compression. If the obstruction is proximal to the probe, then one can expect the dampening of the usual augmentation created by release of proximal compression (Fig. 4-4).

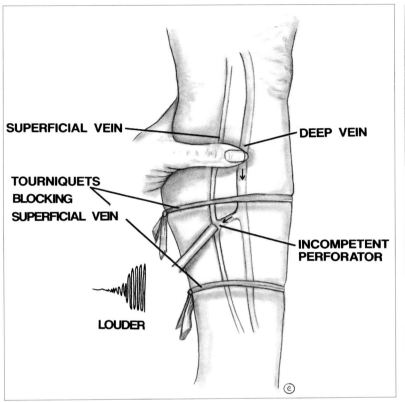

SUPERFICIAL VEIN

DEEP VEIN

TOURNIQUETS
BLOCKING
SUPERFICIAL VEIN

INCOMPETENT
PERFORATOR

LOUDER

A

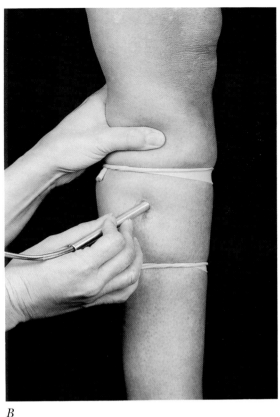

B

Another easy maneuver using the Doppler ultrasound aids in isolating suspected incompetent perforators. A bulging vein at the location of a common perforator or a fascial defect felt when the leg is emptied of blood may lead one to suspect an incompetent perforator at this location. The Doppler ultrasound can be used to confirm the presence of the incompetent perforator. The patient is placed in the supine position and the leg emptied of blood by elevation. Tourniquets are placed proximal and distal to the suspected location to block the flow from the superficial system. Compression proximal to the probe will result in an augmented signal only if there is backflow through an incompetent perforator. Augmentation of the Doppler signal on proximal compression with a tourniquet blocking the superficial system is pathognomonic of an incompetent perforator (Fig. 4–5 and Table 4–3).

FIGURE 4–5. *A,B.*
With tourniquets blocking the superficial system, proximal compression results in an augmented signal only if there is reflux from the deep system through an incompetent perforator.

TABLE 4–3. *Isolation of Incompetent Perforators*
Place tourniquet proximal and distal to probe site to remove superficial system.
Compress proximal to tourniquet.
Augmentation on proximal compression is through incompetent perforator.

The key to successful sclerotherapy is elimination of the point of maximal reflux. The highest point of reflux must first be located. Careful physical examination can rule out significant venous pathology in the patient who clearly has only minor spider veins less than 2 mm in diameter. Some patients may have reticular veins of questionable significance, and in these patients, the Doppler ultrasound is very useful in locating the source of reflux, if any is present. Distal compression over the vein augments the Doppler signal and allows one to trace the vein and determine any connection with the long or short saphenous vein. The lack of augmentation of the signal on the release of distal compression or on proximal compression confirms the lack of significant reflux in the vein. An examination using the inexpensive Doppler ultrasound device that confirms the absence of significant reflux from the saphenous or deep venous system ensures that sclerotherapy can be used effectively.

The Doppler ultrasound examination must be performed with the patient in the standing position because reflux only exists with the leg in the dependent position. The long saphenous vein is examined from the front with the feet turned outward. The short saphenous vein is examined from the back with the knee slightly flexed to avoid possible mechanical obstruction of short saphenous outflow by knee extension.

The presence of reflux in any dilated veins that originate from the saphenous system is certainly significant, and the patient no longer fits the category of spider veins. Reflux in the long or short saphenous system may stem from incompetency at the saphenofemoral or saphenopopliteal junction or from an incompetent perforator. These junctions

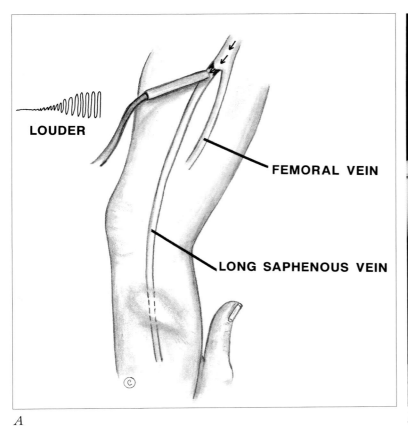

LOUDER

FEMORAL VEIN

LONG SAPHENOUS VEIN

©

A

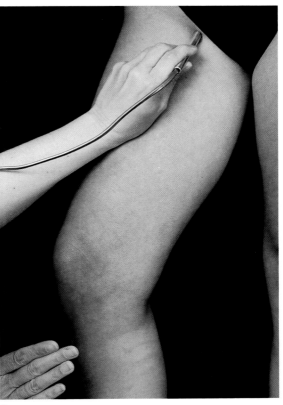

B

FIGURE 4-6. *Reflux at the saphenofemoral junction. A,B. With the probe placed just below the saphenofemoral junction, a loud signal heard for longer than a second on release of distal compression is indicative of reflux.*

can be examined for reflux using the Doppler ultrasound employing the same maneuvers of proximal and distal compression. Reflux is detected on Doppler ultrasound by augmentation of the Doppler signal on release of distal compression and on proximal compression. The Doppler probe is placed just below the saphenofemoral junction. Proximal compression at the saphenofemoral junction can be created by a Valsalva maneuver or cough that applies pressure to the proximal veins. Augmentation of the venous system at the saphenofemoral junction on Valsalva maneuver, which sounds like a prolonged "whoosh," is indicative of incompetency of the valve, the same as augmentation of the venous signal on proximal compression in any other area (Fig. 4–6*E*). Sometimes a short signal may be heard normally prior to the valve

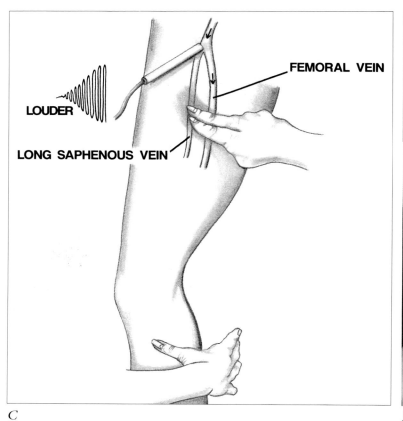

FEMORAL VEIN

LOUDER

LONG SAPHENOUS VEIN

C

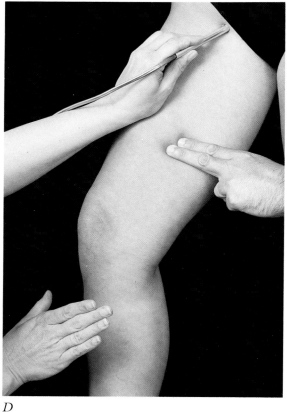

D

FIGURE 4–6. *(Continued) C,D. Repeat the release of distal compression maneuver with fingers obstructing the long saphenous vein. If an augmented signal is still heard, the reflux may be in the femoral vein itself rather than the saphenofemoral junction.*

closing. However, if the "whoosh" lasts longer than a second, it indicates significant reflux. A loud signal heard for longer than a second on release of distal compression is indicative of reflux (Fig. 4–6*A,B*). In order to distinguish reflux in the long saphenous vein originating at the saphenofemoral junction rather than in the femoral vein itself, one can repeat this maneuver of released distal compression with fingers obstructing the long saphenous vein in the vicinity of the junction. If augmentation of the signal on release of distal compression indicative of reflux is still heard, the reflux signal may be stemming from the femoral vein rather than the saphenofemoral junction (Fig. 4–6*C,D*).

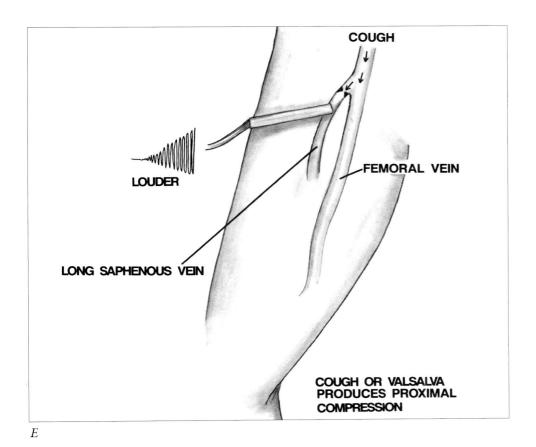

E

FIGURE 4–6. *(Continued)* *E. A loud signal lasting longer than a second at the saphenofemoral junction produced by coughing or a Valsalva maneuver (proximal compression) confirms the presence of reflux.*

These same maneuvers to determine reflux can then be performed in the popliteal fossa in order to determine if reflux is present at the saphenopopliteal junction. With the patient standing with the knee slightly flexed, the popliteal arterial signal is located just above the knee flexion creases. The venous signal is then located just lateral to the arterial signal. This venous signal is easily found by distally compressing the leg in order to augment the venous flow. On release of distal compression, if reflux is detected with augmentation of the Doppler signal, then this may represent reflux in the popliteal vein or in the short saphenous vein stemming from the saphenopopliteal junction. In order to locate the site of the reflux, a finger is placed obstructing the short saphenous vein. The release of distal compression is repeated. If an

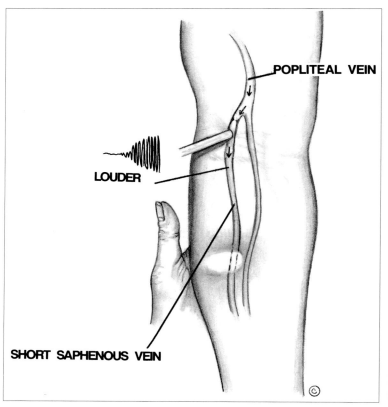

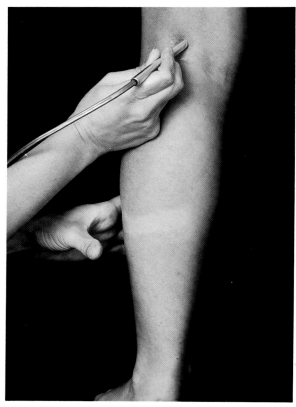

POPLITEAL VEIN

LOUDER

SHORT SAPHENOUS VEIN

A

B

FIGURE 4–7. *Reflux at the saphenopopliteal junction. A,B. With the probe placed just below the saphenopopliteal junction, a loud signal heard on release of distal compression is indicative of reflux. C,D. Repeat the release of distal compression maneuver with fingers obstructing the short saphenous vein. If an augmented signal is still heard, the reflux may be in the popliteal vein itself rather than the saphenopopliteal junction. E,F. A loud signal heard at the saphenopopliteal junction with proximal compression confirms the presence of reflux.*

augmented Doppler signal is still present, indicative of reflux, then this may represent reflux in the popliteal vein rather than the short saphenous vein. If it is obliterated, then the reflux is in the short saphenous vein stemming from the saphenopopliteal junction. Finally, the reflux can be confirmed by the additional maneuver of proximal compression, which also exacerbates the reflux, if present, augmenting the venous signal. (Fig. 4–7 *A-F*).

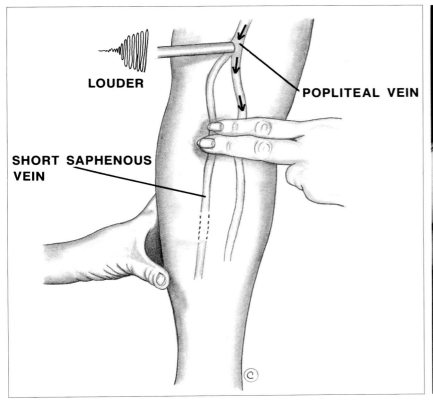

LOUDER

POPLITEAL VEIN

SHORT SAPHENOUS
VEIN

C

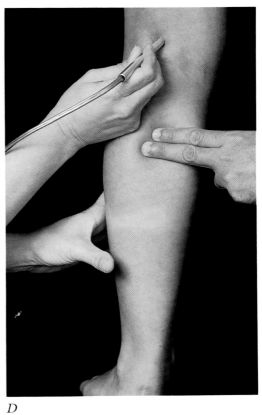

D

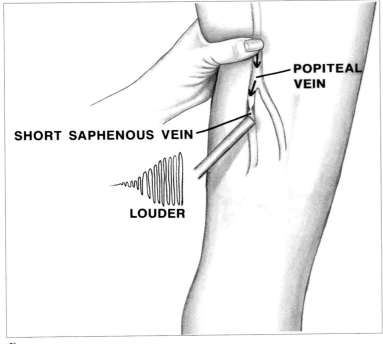

POPITEAL
VEIN

SHORT SAPHENOUS VEIN

LOUDER

E

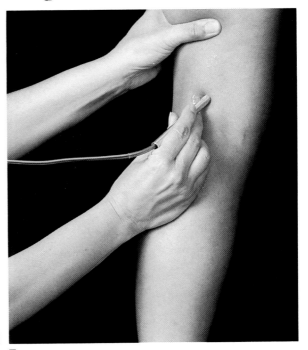

F

FIGURE 4–7. *(Continued)*

T A B L E 4–4. *Acute Deep Venous Thrombosis*
Dampened augmentation on distal compression if obstruction distally. Dampened augmentation on release of proximal compression if obstruction proximally.

Reflux of this magnitude which stems from the junction or results in large dilatations of the saphenous systems or their tributaries may require operative management, and the treatment differs significantly from that for spider veins. The Doppler ultrasound is a useful tool to rule out major reflux in the saphenous system in order to distinguish these patients from the huge population of patients who suffer from spider veins alone.

The Doppler ultrasound also can be used to detect venous obstruction secondary to thrombosis. The maneuvers of distal compression and release of proximal compression that normally augment the venous system result in a dampened Doppler signal when the flow is obstructed (Table 4–4). Acute deep vein thrombosis is often apparent clinically as

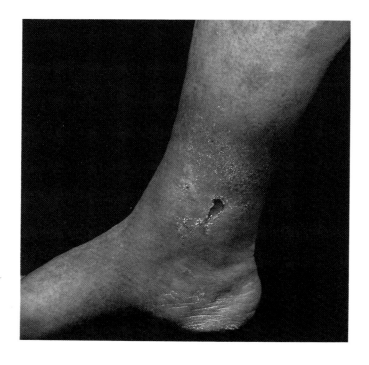

FIGURE 4–8.
Postphlebitic syndrome. The presence of brawny edema, stasis dermatitis, or ulceration warrants an extensive venous evaluation.

TABLE 4–5. *Locations to Examine Deep Veins*

Posterial Tibial Vein: Posterior to Medial Malleolous
Popliteal Vein: Popiteal Fossa
Superficial Femoral Vein: Mid-Thigh
Common Femoral Vein: Just Below Inguinal Ligament
Identify Accompanying Arterial Signal First, Then Venous Signal.

unilateral leg swelling and calf tenderness. The postphlebitic syndrome, which can occur as a late manifestation of venous thrombosis, is hallmarked clinically by brawny edema, dermatitis, and ulceration (Fig. 4–8). These patients must have an extensive evaluation of the deep venous system. In order to locate the deep veins by Doppler ultrasound, the accompanying arterial signal is first identified and then the adjacent venous signal. The posterior tibial vein is examined posterior to the medial malleolus, the popliteal vein in the popliteal fossa, the superficial femoral vein at midthigh level, and the common femoral vein just below the inguinal ligament (Table 4–5).

Patients with venous thrombosis and chronic venous insufficiency require extensive evaluation of their underlying venous pathology. Clinical examination and Doppler ultrasound can be used quite effectively to distinguish these patients from those who suffer from spider veins alone.

LIGHT REFLECTION RHEOGRAPHY (LRR)

Another screening tool for patients with spider veins is light reflection rheography. This is another method of noninvasive examination of the venous system that can screen patients with spider veins to rule out venous obstruction or significant reflux. This method provides hemodynamic information about venous outflow rather than an anatomic visualization of the venous system.

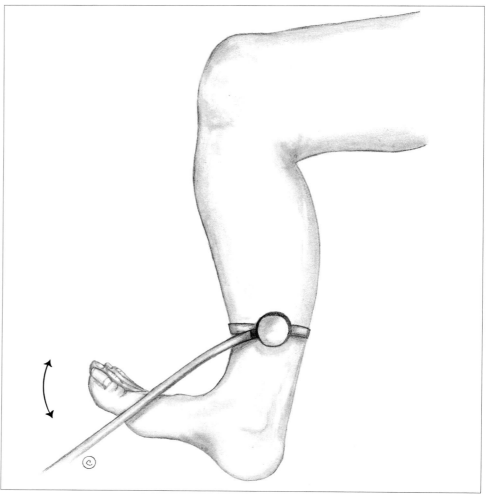

A

FIGURE 4–9. *Light reflection rheography (LRR). A. After an infrared sensor is taped on the leg 10.0 cm above the medial malleolus, the patient performs 10 rhythmic dorsiflexions of the foot, activating the calf muscle pump and propelling the blood back to the heart. B. The LRR machine plots a graph of the venous outflow during the dorsiflexions and the following venous inflow.*

An infrared sensor is taped on the leg 10 cm above the medial malleolus. The patient performs 10 rhythmic dorsiflexions of the foot (Fig. 4–9).

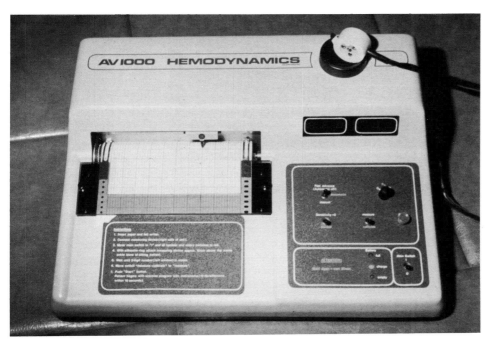

B

F I G U R E 4–9. *(Continued)*

These movements activate the calf muscle pump, which propels the blood back to the heart. The LRR machine plots a graph of the venous outflow during exercise, and the following venous refilling time is measured. Normal refilling time is 25 seconds. Rapid refilling in less than 25 seconds indicates venous insufficiency. Tourniquets are then used to eliminate the contribution of the superficial venous system. Normalization of the refilling time with tourniquets in place indicates superficial venous insufficiency; no improvement is suggestive of deep venous insufficiency.[2] A flattened outflow curve depicting poor outflow with rapid refilling time is suggestive of deep venous thrombosis.

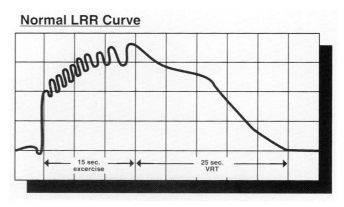

Normal LRR Curve

A

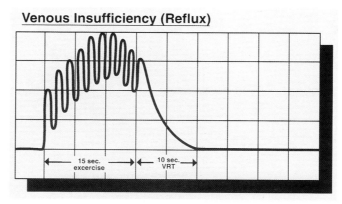

Venous Insufficiency (Reflux)

B

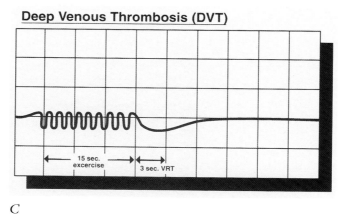

Deep Venous Thrombosis (DVT)

C

FIGURE 4–10. *A. Normal LRR curve showing venous emptying with exercise and normal venous refilling time (VRT = 25 sec.). B. Rapid venous refilling indicates reflux. C. Flattened curve showing poor venous outflow and rapid refill is suggestive of deep venous thrombosis.*

The LRR unit (Fig. 4–10) costs approximately $4500 compared with $575 for a Doppler ultrasound device. The patient interested in sclerotherapy of cosmetic spider veins is very concerned about the total cost necessary to obtain the desired cosmetic results. Both methods of examination of the venous system allow one to assess the presence of reflux and obstruction in the major venous system. Although LRR provides more information about the volume of reflux, the Doppler ultrasound allows more direct assessment of the source of reflux, particularly in cases of minor reflux.

LRR is a form of photoplethysmography (PPG), i.e., a measurement of the changes in blood volume accomplished by light. The air plethysmograph uses an air cuff to quantitate venous outflow, venous reflux, and calf pump function. Air plethysmography provides invaluable quantitative data on venous hemodynamics noninvasively. This information is important for evaluating patients with chronic deep venous insufficiency; however, it is superfluous in cases of spider veins and minor isolated reflux.

DUPLEX SCANNING

Duplex scanning combines the hemodynamic evaluation made with the Doppler ultrasound with an anatomic visualization of the vein provided by B-mode real-time ultrasound with a 5– to 10–MHz imaging probe. The anatomic imaging of the vein being evaluated hemodynamically for reflux or obstruction eliminates the anatomic uncertainty inherent in the Doppler ultrasound alone. The user actually sees the vein lumen, the venous valves, the blood flow in color, and the thrombi in the lumen of the veins, in addition to simultaneously hearing the Doppler signal change with the maneuvers of distal and proximal compression or release (Fig. 4–11).

This allows the practitioner to precisely locate the sites of reflux and obstruction. The precise anatomic localization of the source of reflux ensures exact placement of the sclerosing agent at the source of reflux for optimal sclerotherapy results. This is quite helpful in sclerotherapy of major venous trunks and at the saphenofemoral and saphenopopliteal junctions. However, it provides more detail than is usually necessary for successful sclerotherapy of spider veins. The duplex

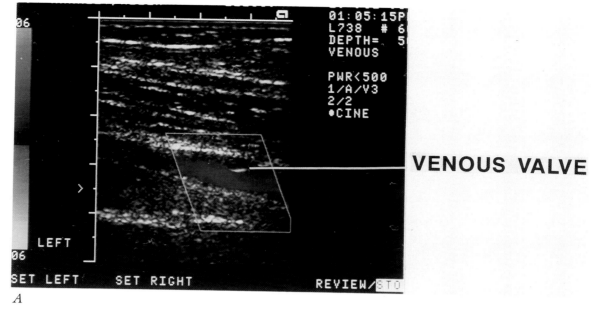

VENOUS VALVE

THROMBUS

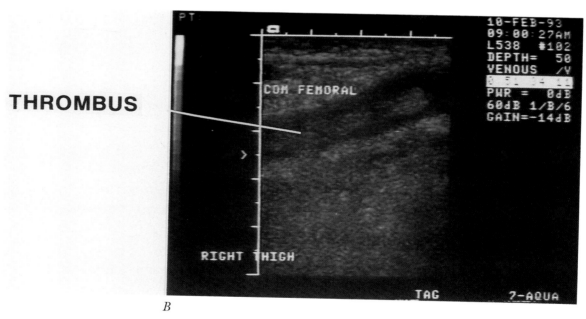

FIGURE 4-11. *Duplex scanning. A. A duplex scan combines the Doppler ultrasound with anatomic venous imaging, showing the vein lumen, blood flow in color, and venous valves. B. Thrombi in the vein lumen also can be seen on a duplex scan.*

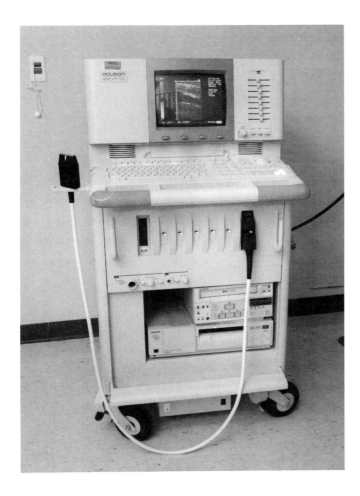

FIGURE 4–12. *The duplex scanner is large, cumbersome, and unnecessarily expensive for the practice of sclerotherapy of spider veins alone.*

scanner itself is large, cumbersome, and expensive at approximately $150,000, especially when compared with the Doppler ultrasound (Fig. 4–12).

REFERENCES

1. Thibault PK, Lewis WA. Recurrent varicose veins Part 1: Evaluation utilizing duplex venous imaging. J Dermatol Surg Oncol 1992; 18: 618–624.
2. O'Donnell TF Jr, McEnroe CS, Heggerick P. Chronic venous insufficiency. Surg Clin North Am 1990; 70: 159–166.

ADDITIONAL READINGS

Doppler Ultrasound

Barnes RW, Russell HE, Wu KK, et al. Accuracy of Doppler ultrasound in clinically suspected venous thrombosis of the calf. Surg Gynecol Obstet 1976; 143:425–428.

Barnes RW, Ross EA, Strandness DE Jr. Differentiation of primary from secondary varicose veins by Doppler ultrasound and strain gauge plethysmography. Surg Gynecol Obstet 1975; 141:207–211.

Barnes RW, Russell HE, Wilson MR. Doppler Ultrasonic Evaluation of Venous Disease: A Programmed Audiovisual Instruction, 2d ed. Iowa City: University of Iowa Press, 1975.

Barnes RW. Doppler ultrasonic diagnosis of venous disease. In Bernstein EF, ed: Noninvasive Diagnostic Techniques in Vascular Disease, 3d ed. St. Louis: Mosby, 1985, pp 724–729.

Evans DS, Cockett FB. Diagnosis of deep-vein thrombosis with an ultrasonic Doppler technique. Br Med J 1969; 2:802–804.

Folse R, Alexander RH. Directional flow detection for localizing venous valvular incompetency. Surgery 1970; 67:114–121.

Foote AV, Miller SS. Ultrasonic flow probe detection of incompetent perforating veins. Scott Med J 1969; 14:96.

Raju S, Fredericks R. Evaluation of methods for detecting venous reflux: Perspectives in venous insufficiency. Arch Surg 1990; 125:1463–1467.

Schultz-Ehrenburg U, Hübner H-J. Reflux Diagnosis with Doppler Ultrasound (Monograph). Stuttgart: Schattauer, 1989.

Sigel B, Popky GL, Boland JP, et al. Diagnosis of venous disease by ultrasonic flow detection. Surg Forum 1967; 18:185–187.

Sigel B, Popky GL, Wagner DK, et al. Comparison of clinical and Doppler ultrasound evaluation of confirmed lower extremity venous disease. Surgery 1968; 64:332–338.

Sigel B, Popky GL, Wagner DK, et al. A Doppler ultrasound method for diagnosing lower extremity venous disease. Surg Gynecol Obstet 1968; 127:339–350.

Sigel B, Popky GL, Mapp EM, et al. Evaluation of Doppler ultrasound examination. Arch Surg 1970; 100:535–540.

Sumner DS, Lambeth A. Reliability of Doppler ultrasound in the diagnosis of acute venous thrombosis both above and below the knee. Am J Surg 1979; 138:205–210.

Photoplethysmography

Nicolaides AN, Miles C. Photoplethysmography in the assessment of venous insufficiency. J Vasc Surg 1987; 5:405–412.

Norris CS, Beyrau A, Barnes RW. Quantitative photoplethysmography in chronic venous insufficiency: A new method of noninvasive estimation of ambulatory venous pressure. Surgery 1983; 94:758–764.

Sarin S, Shields DA, Scurr JH, Smith PDC. Photoplethysmography: A valuable noninvasive tool in the assessment of venous dysfunction? J Vasc Surg 1992; 16:154–162.

Duplex Scanning

Quigley FG, Raptis S, Cashman M, Faris IB. Duplex ultrasound mapping of sites of deep to superficial incompetence in primary varicose veins. Aust NZ J Med 1992; 62:276–278.

Rosfors S, Bygdeman S, Nordström E. Assessment of deep venous incompetence: A prospective study comparing duplex scanning with descending phlebography. Angiology 1990; 41:463–468.

Szendro G, Nicolaides AN, Zukowski AJ, et al. Duplex scanning in the assessment of deep venous incompetence. J Vasc Surg 1986; 4:237–242.

Vasdekis SN, Clarke GH, Nicolaides AN. Quantification of venous reflux by means of duplex scanning. J Vasc Surg 1989; 10:670–677.

SCLEROSING AGENTS

5

AFTER THE PATIENT has been properly evaluated as a candidate for sclerotherapy, the next step is the choice of the sclerosing agent and concentration. Some practitioners use only one agent exclusively for sclerotherapy of spider veins. A more flexible attitude and experience with several different agents allows a choice of the best agent for the particular patient based on a thorough history and physical examination.

MECHANISM OF ACTION

Many sclerosing agents have been used since the 1800s for the treatment of such diverse conditions as recurrent pleural effusions, ganglions, hernias, esophageal varices, and hemorrhoids, as well as varicose veins and spider veins.[1] Sclerosing agents basically are irritants that injure the endothelial surfaces, ultimately resulting in obliteration of the space between these surfaces.[2] Sclerosing agents are classified into three groups based on the mechanism of action causing the injury to the endothelium: the *detergents*, including polidocanol, sodium tetradecyl sulfate, and sodium morrhuate; the *osmotics*, including hypertonic saline and hypertonic saline-dextrose; and the *chemical irritants*, including chromated glycerin.[3]

The detergents cause injury by altering the surface tension surrounding the cells. The osmotic agents cause injury by dehydrating the

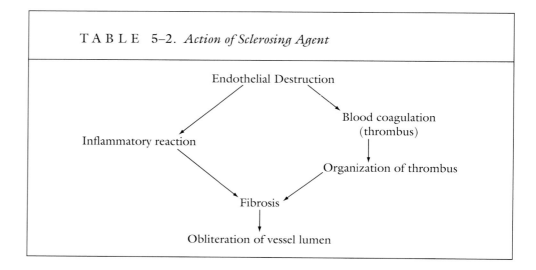

TABLE 5-1. *Mechanism of Action of Sclerosing Agents*

1. Detergents
   A. Polidocanol
   B. Sodium tetradecyl sulfate
   C. Sodium morrhuate
2. Osmotic agents
   A. Hypertonic saline
   B. Hypertonic saline-dextrose
3. Chemical irritants
   A. Chromated glycerin
   B. Polyiodinated iodide

TABLE 5-2. *Action of Sclerosing Agent*

Endothelial Destruction

Inflammatory reaction

Blood coagulation (thrombus)

Organization of thrombus

Fibrosis

Obliteration of vessel lumen

endothelial cells. The chemical irritants include the corrosives, which act by a cauterizing action, and those which injure cells by a heavy metal effect (Table 5–1). The destruction of the endothelium elicits an inflammatory reaction as well as activation of the intrinsic clotting pathway leading to thrombus formation.[4,5] The result of this reaction and organization of the thrombus is fibrosis with obliteration of the vessel lumen (Table 5–2).

Large thrombi are frequently recanalized, leading to a higher rate of recurrence. Optimally, then, this fibrosis occurs following as little thrombus formation as possible.[2,6]

it is impossible for it to elicit an allergic reaction. It is possible that lidocaine also may be free of documented hypersensitivity.[32,33] Although some authors would dispute this, it is a consensus of opinion that an anaphylactic reaction to lidocaine is extraordinarily rare for such a commonly used anesthetic agent.[34] However, the 2% lidocaine hydrochloride commonly used for dilutions comes in a multidose vial under the trademark Xylocaine, and it contains 1 mg methylparaben as an antiseptic preservative. Rare cases of allergic reaction have been traced to this preservative. Lidocaine 2% is also readily available without this preservative.

The only limit on the maximal amount of hypertonic saline that can be used at a single treatment session is governed by the maximal amount of salt intake that can be tolerated by the individual patient. Even in a case of extensive spider vein involvement, one would seldom find a need to exceed 10 cc of a sclerosing agent. This would amount to 1.87 g salt if 10 cc of the 18.7% solution were used. This amount should be easily tolerated by any patient without a history of congestive heart failure.

Certainly, there is a strict limit on the amount of lidocaine that can be injected at a single treatment session. Toxic doses of lidocaine can result in convulsions and cardiovascular depression and arrest.* Intravenously, this dose should not exceed 4.5 mg/kg in adults. This is equivalent to 15 cc of 2% lidocaine in a 70-kg adult. This amount exceeds several times the amount that would maximally be needed as the diluent in a single session, even in cases of extensive spider vein involvement.

Hypertonic saline 23.4% will cause skin ulceration if injected perivascularly. The rates of the most common complications of sclerotherapy of spider veins are acceptably low with the use of hypertonic saline as the sclerosing agent, particularly if diluted to less than 20%. Decreasing the concentration of hypertonic saline decreases the complication rate. One study reported effective vein sclerosis of vessels less than 8 mm in

*Package insert, Xylocaine, Elkins-Sinn, Inc., Cherry Hill, NJ 08003-4099.

diameter with as a low as 11.7% hypertonic saline diluted with normal saline or heparin.[31] However, the mean number of treatments required to effectively sclerose a vein in this study was 3.5 at 4-week intervals.

Polidocanol

Polidocanol was first developed for possible use as an anesthetic agent; however, this use was abandoned when sclerosing properties were noted.[35] It since has been used widely in Europe for sclerotherapy of smaller veins.

The active agent is hydroxypolyaethoxydodecan. The most common trade name is Aethoxysklerol (Kreussler & Co., Germany). It is also trademarked as Sclerovein (Vascular Products, Inc., England). Polidocanol is not yet FDA approved, but clinical trials for FDA approval are ongoing. Pending the results of these clinical trials, FDA approval is anticipated.

The mechanism of action of polidocanol as a sclerosing agent is that of a detergent, weaker in strength than sodium tetradecyl sulfate. It has been used in concentrations of 2% to 3% for sclerotherapy of large varices. However, since it is a weak detergent, its strength as a sclerosing agent has been insufficient for the treatment of larger varices.[36] It is much more widely used for sclerotherapy of spider veins in concentrations of 0.25% to 0.75%. In one study, the 0.5% solution was found to be most effective with fewer complications, making it the optimal concentration for sclerotherapy of spider veins.[37]

Polidocanol is available from Europe in 30-ml vials and 2-ml ampules of 0.5%, 1%, 2%, and 3% solutions. Common formulas for dilution of polidocanol for use in sclerotherapy of spider veins are found in Table 5–3. A daily dose of 2 mg/kg of body weight should not be exceeded.* This dose is equivalent to 28 cc of the 0.5% solution in a 70-kg person, which well exceeds the usual amount that would be

*Package insert, Aethoxysklerol, Kreussler Pharma Chemische Fabrik, Kreussler & Co., GmbH D-6200 Wiesbaden-Biebrich.

required for a single treatment session, even in the case of extensive spider vein involvement.

Consistent with its original development as an anesthetic agent, polidocanol is virtually painless on injection at weaker concentrations.[29,37-39] Temporary itching may occur following injection.[37] It is a well-tolerated sclerosing agent with a low incidence of complications and rare allergic reactions. Its most outstanding advantage in sclerotherapy of spider veins is the very low rate of ulceration on perivascular infiltration of weak concentrations. In fact, 0.5% polidocanol has been deliberately injected intradermally around tiny telangiectasias that could not be entered intravascularly without producing skin necrosis.[40] This technique of perivascular infiltration is not advocated, however, and higher concentrations can produce limited necrosis.[26,41] The rates of hyperpigmentation and telangiectatic matting are also relatively low.

Serious allergic reactions to polidocanol are extremely rare at 0.01% to 0.02% and there has been only one reported case of an anaphylactic reaction.[4,37,42,43] Polidocanol has been used in patients who are allergic to other sclerosants such as sodium tetradecyl sulfate.[36] There are two relative contraindications particular to the sclerosing agent polidocanol noted by the manufacturer. Bronchial asthma is one relative contraindication.* Another is during or after alcohol withdrawal treatment with agents such as Disulfiram because a small amount of absolute ethyl alcohol is added to polidocanol to furnish heat stability.

The results obtained using polidocanol for sclerotherapy of spider veins can be dramatic. However, the process of sclerosis is slower than with the stronger detergent sodium tetradecyl sulfate or even hypertonic saline.[29] Patients must be warned that they will only see approximately 50 to 70 percent lightening of the spider veins after the first few treatment sessions (Fig. 5–2). Between 4 and 6 weeks are usually allowed between treatment sessions for sclerosis to occur with polidocanol, and two to six treatments may be necessary on each spider vein for optimal sclerosing.[29,42]

*Package insert, Aethoxysklerol, Kreussler Pharma Chemische Fabrik, Kreussler & Co., GmbH D-6200 Wiesbaden-Biebrich.

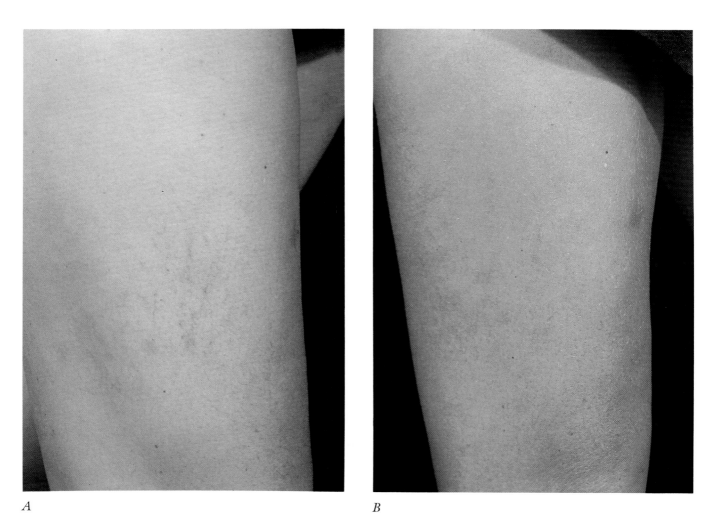

A
B

FIGURE 5–2. *A. Before sclerotherapy. B. Four weeks after one sclerotherapy treatment with 0.5% polidocanol showing the degree of lightening that can be expected after a single injection. C. Four weeks after second treatment. Even in cases of such minor spider veins as these, a second treatment achieves even further obliteration.*

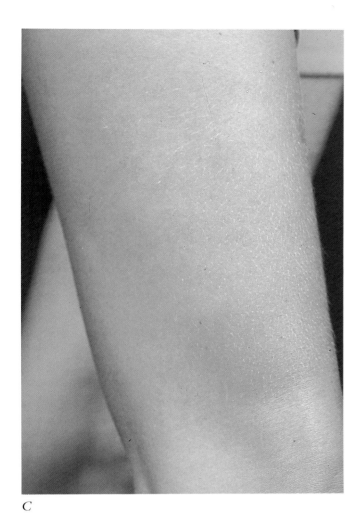

C

FIGURE 5–2. *(Continued)*

Sodium Morrhuate

Sodium morrhuate is a complex mixture of fatty acids that is essentially a cod liver oil extract. It has been used for sclerotherapy of varicose veins since it was first prepared in the 1920s by Ghosh[44] and Cutting.[45] The trade name is Scleromate. It is a strong detergent. It is FDA approved and is widely available in the United States in 30-ml multi-use vials of 5% from Palisades Pharmaceuticals, Inc.

Sodium morrhuate has been used extensively in the past for sclerotherapy of varicose veins. It also has been used for sclerotherapy of spider veins in dilute solutions ranging from 0.25% to 0.5%. One of the earlier pioneers of sclerotherapy of spider veins, H. I. Biegeleisen, reported his experience with sodium morrhuate for this purpose as early as 1934.[46] Although it still has a few proponents, most practitioners have abandoned the use of sodium morrhuate, even in dilute concentrations, for sclerotherapy of spider veins.[47] One of the main reasons is the high rate of ulceration with perivascular infiltration, even in dilute concentrations. Another disadvantage to using sodium morrhuate is the variety of allergic reactions that have been reported, ranging from such mild reactions as urticaria to asthma, respiratory depression, gastrointestinal disturbances such as nausea and vomiting, vascular collapse, and anaphylaxis.[48-51]

Hypertonic Glucose-Saline

Hypertonic glucose-saline solutions have been used for sclerotherapy of varicose veins since 1929 as reported by Kern and Angle.[21] A hypertonic glucose-saline solution known under the trade name Sclerodex is commonly used in Canada for sclerotherapy of spider veins. Sclerodex contains 25% dextrose and 10% sodium chloride in 0.8% phenethyl alcohol as local anesthetic.[17] The mechanism of action is dehydration by osmosis, similar to hypertonic saline. It is a very mild sclerosing agent. It is not FDA approved, is produced by Laboratoire Ondee, Ltd., in Montreal, and is available in 10-cc ampules from Omega in Montreal, Canada.

Since Sclerodex is a weak sclerosing agent, it is used primarily on spider veins and small-caliber reticular veins. It usually does not require dilution; however, it can be diluted with a small volume of saline solution (4:1). In Canada, it is sometimes mixed with small amounts of polyiodinated iodine (Sclerodine) to increase its sclerosing power.

There is minimal pain on injection of Sclerodex. The maximum amount recommended for injection in any single treatment session is 10 cc, according to the manufacturer.

Mantse[17] has used this agent in more than 500 patients and reports a very low rate of complications (such as hyperpigmentation 0.6%, superficial skin necrosis 0.2%, and telangiectatic matting 0.4%). It is important to note, however, that these rates represent the use of this agent for only very tiny telangiectasias on the medial aspect of the thighs, since it is such a weak sclerosing agent. Mantse also noted only one allergic reaction, for a rate of 0.2%.

Chromated Glycerin

Jausion used chromated glycerin as a sclerosing agent as early as 1925.[52] It is now popular in Europe for sclerotherapy of spiders veins and is marketed under the trade name Scleremo. Scleremo is composed of 72% chromated glycerin. The mechanism of action is that of a chemical irritant. It is a very mild sclerosing agent. It is not FDA approved, nor is it anticipated to seek FDA approval in the near future. It is produced by Laboratoires E. Bauteille in France and available in 5–ml vials.

Since chromated glycerin is such a weak sclerosing agent, its use is limited to spider veins and small-caliber reticular veins.[53] It has a high viscosity, so it is usually diluted 1:1 to 4:1 with saline or 1% lidocaine.

Chromated glycerin does cause some local pain as well as occasional cramps in remote areas. This can be minimized with the use of lidocaine as the diluent. It is particularly painful on extravenous extravasation.

Chromated glycerin has a low incidence of side effects. Allergic reactions are very rare.[54] Postsclerotherapy pigmentation and cutaneous necrosis are extremely rare, and these are the primary advantages of this sclerosing agent.[55] Because chromated glycerin has a lower rate of pigmentation than polidocanol, Georgiev[56] recommends a trial of chromated glycerin on patients with spider and reticular veins alone. If patients do not respond to the weaker chromated glycerin with sufficient reaction to predict effective sclerosis in a reasonable number of treatment sessions, only then would he recommend changing agents to the stronger polidocanol.

TABLE 5–4. Summary of Sclerosing Agents

Generic Name	Common Trade Names	Concentrations Commonly Used for Spider Veins	Pain	Mechanism of Action	Relative Strength of Agent	FDA Approved	Allergic Reactions	Maximal Amount for Each Session	Incidence of Ulceration
Sodium tetradecyl sulfate	Sotradecol (U.S.) Thrombovar (Europe)	0.33% (0.1–0.5%)	minimal	detergent	2	yes	rare	10 cc of 1% or 3%	infrequent
Hypertonic saline		18.7% with 0.4% lidocaine (11.7%–23.4%) may be diluted with heparin or saline	yes (unless diluted with lidocaine)	dehydration by osmosis	3	yes, but only as abortifacient	none	only limited by salt intake	rare when diluted
Polidocanol	Aethoxysklerol Sclerovein	0.5% (0.25%–0.75%)	none	detergent	5	no (in clinical trials)	vary rare	2mg/kg	very rare
Sodium morrhuate	Scleromate	0.25%–0.5%	yes	detergent	1	yes	yes	not determined	most frequent
Hypertonic glucose/saline	Sclerodex	usually undiluted	minimal	dehydration by osmosis	4	no	very rare	10cc	rare
Chromated glycerin	Scleremo	usually diluted 1:1 or 4:1 with saline or 1% lidocaine	yes (unless diluted with lidocaine)	chemical irritant	6	no	very rare	10 cc	extremely rare

6

INJECTION TECHNIQUE

PATIENT PREPARATION

Informed Consent

The most important factor in patient preparation is patient education. This can begin effectively as the patient signs in for the appointment. The receptionist can then give the patient an information sheet on the procedure for the patient to read while waiting to be seen. A sample instruction sheet for sclerotherapy of spider veins is provided in Table 6–1. After the history and physical examination, a treatment plan is formulated for the patient. A frank discussion about all aspects of the procedure is necessary for informed consent. The aesthetic goals are discussed, as well as the limitations of the procedure, in order to provide the patient with realistic expectations. The possible complications, the alternatives of treatment, the normal recovery period, the postprocedure care and restrictions, the approximate time required to complete the treatment plan, and the cost must all be addressed prior to beginning sclerotherapy. For the sake of instructional continuity, these are the subjects of later chapters. However, the cosmetic patient needs to know all this information prior to the first injections so as to give informed consent and to fit the treatment protocol into his or her schedule. A sample sclerotherapy consent form is provided in Table 6–2.

TABLE 6–1. *Spider Vein Injections*

PATIENT INFORMATION

Sclerotherapy of spider veins is a procedure designed to decrease the visibility of unsightly spider veins commonly found on legs and occasionally on other areas. The procedure involves the injection of a medication into each of the involved veins that "closes" the vein so that it no longer is visible. We have found patient satisfaction with the procedure to be high as long as patients understand all the following important information about the procedure. All of these points will be addressed at your consultation, and we welcome any questions you may have.

1. The treatment of spider veins of the lower extremities will require more than one series of injections, as will be determined in your initial consultation.

2. The injections are performed with you lying down. You will feel some slight discomfort from the fine needle sticks, the number of which will be determined by the number of veins requiring treatment. The medicine may cause mild discomfort on injection.

3. There have been reported rare cases of allergic reactions to the medication. Do not hesitate to tell us if you feel faint or have any discomfort during your treatment.

4. The average treatment session takes approximately 30 minutes.

5. A compressive dressing will be applied to the injection sites. You should leave this dressing on for 48 hours.

6. You may feel some cramping in your legs for the first day or two after the injections.

7. The veins will look worse before they look better. By this we mean that there will be some bruising at the injection sites that will decrease over approximately one month's time. In many cases, there may be some residual brownish pigmentation that gradually fades over a period of approximately one year.

8. In rare cases, the skin overlying the vein can be injured resulting in a wound which on healing will leave a scar.

9. If you notice blue-black clots in the treated veins after the tapes are removed, please call the office.

10. Follow-up will usually consist of monthly visits until the treatment plan is completed.

11. The doctor may wrap your legs or give you a prescription for compressive stockings to be worn after your treatment, if necessary.

12. Please DO NOT apply moisturizer or other creams to your legs on the day of your injections.

13. Walking is encouraged after the injections.

14. Avoid prolonged sitting and standing, pounding-type exercises, squatting, and heavy weight lifting after the injections.

TABLE 6-2. *Consent to Sclerotherapy of Spider Veins*

Patient:_____

Date of procedure:_____

I hereby authorize Dr. _____ to perform a procedure upon me
known as: <u>Spider Vein Injections</u>.

1. I hereby give permission to take photographs that may be used for medical
   publication, education, or records, provided my identity is not revealed.

2. The details of the procedure listed above have been explained to me and I
   understand the nature and consequence of the procedure. Alternative methods
   of treatment, including laser therapy, cauterization, and phlebectomy, have
   been explained to me as have the advantages and disadvantages of each. The
   following points have been specifically made clear:

a. The possible complications, including scars, pigment changes, clots in veins,
   appearance of fine red blood vessels, and allergic reactions, have all been
   explained to me.

b. The limitations of the procedure have been discussed, including the possible
   reoccurrence or occurrence of new spider veins in the future.

c. The practice of medicine and surgery is not an exact science and that, therefore,
   reputable practitioners cannot properly guarantee results either expressed or
   implied.

3. I authorize the operating surgeon to perform any other procedure that he/she
   may deem necessary or desirable in attempting to improve the condition as
   stated in the above procedure or any other unhealthy or unforseen condition
   he/she may encounter during the operation.

4. I hereby give permission for my blood to be drawn for HIV testing in the event
   that the physician or any other health care worker has a significant exposure
   incident (i.e., blood in eye, needle stick, etc.) during my procedure.

5. I consent to the administration of anesthetics to be applied by or under the
   direction of _____ and to the use of such anesthetics as he/
   she may deem advisable in my case with the exception of _____.

6. I am not known to be allergic to anything except _____.

7. I have read the above carefully and fully understand the same and do authorize
   the above physician to perform this procedure on me.

Patient _____

Witness _____

Date _____

Preoperative Instructions

The patient should be instructed to avoid all leg creams for 24 hours prior to the injections. The patient may need to purchase support stockings prior to proceeding with the injections depending on the severity of the spider veins present. The patient should bring shorts to wear for the injections and a long skirt or loose pants to cover the tapes after the injections.

The first injections can be performed during the same visit as the initial consultation if the patient has been properly prepared in advance. Scheduling the injections at another visit usually is more efficient and easier for both patient and physician.

Photography

After the patient has changed into shorts for the injections, the legs are photographed for the permanent record. The lighting must be optimal for the spider veins to show up adequately on the slides. It is difficult to standardize the views because patients differ in the number of spider veins and the locations involved. However, inclusion of a recognizable joint such as a portion of the knee or ankle helps tremendously in orienting the picture for later use. Use of the pretreatment slides as a guide for duplication in the posttreatment slides also aids in standardization and in accurate comparisons.

The sclerotherapy consent form can include consent for taking and using photographs, although a second consent for the photography also may be used (Table 6–3).

MATERIALS

The materials required to practice sclerotherapy of spider veins are relatively inexpensive and easy to obtain. Many of the items are used in all medical specialties and are commonplace in offices of all types of physicians. The basic supplies needed for sclerotherapy of spider veins are listed below, and some of the specialty suppliers are listed in Table 6–4.

Patient:_____ Date_____

    In connection with the medical services which I am receiving from my physician, _____, I consent that clinical photographs may be taken of me or parts of my body under the following conditions:

1. The photographs may be taken only with the consent of my physician and under such conditions and at such times as may be approved by him.
2. The photographs shall be taken by my physician or by a photographer approved by my physician.
3. The photographs shall be used for medical record purposes and shall remain the property of my physician.
4. The photographs shall be used for medical records, and if in the judgement of my physician, medical research, education or science will be benefited by their use, such photographs and information relating to my case may be published and republished, either separately or in connection with each other, in professional journals or medical books, or used for any other purpose that my physician may deem proper in the interest of medical education, knowledge, or research, provided, however, that it is specifically understood that in any such publication or use I shall not be identified by name.

Patient's Signature _____

Parent's Signature _____

Date _____

Witness_____

1. Camera with 105–mm macro lens and flash
2. Black photography background, at least floor length
3. Electric table or examination table
4. Stool (rolling)
5. Mayo stand or counter top
6. Movable overhead spotlights or portable light
7. Magnifying glasses (X2), focal distance 18 in, or magnifying loupes or visor
8. Sclerosing agents
9. Plastic or glass syringes, 1 and 3 cc

10. 30–gauge 1/2–in needles for injection

11. Larger (approximately 20–gauge) needle for making dilutions

12. 25–gauge butterfly needles

13. Needle depository

14. Gloves

15. Bacteriostatic normal saline

16. 2% plain Xylocaine for dilution of hypertonic saline

17. Alcohol

18. Cotton balls

19. Elastic tape

20. 1–in paper tape

21. Compressive leg wrap or stockings

22. Storage box for supplies

23. Lancets, no. 11 blades, or 25–gauge needles for evacuating thrombi

TECHNICAL DETAILS

The injections are performed with the patient lying down. An examination table will suffice; however, an electric table allows the practitioner to adjust the height of the table to a comfortable level while injecting. Sclerotherapy of spider veins is very tedious, so comfort both for the practitioner and the patient is important. The injections are easily performed with the practitioner sitting on the stool. A rolling stool is preferred because it allows quick changes of position to access all the areas requiring injections. The supplies are laid out on a counter top or preferably on a rolling Mayo stand. A model tray setup for sclerotherapy includes all supplies needed: alcohol, sclerosing agent, needles, syringes, magnification glasses, tape, cotton balls, and elastic compression bandage. This Mayo stand can easily be rolled to follow the practitioner around the legs as the injections proceed. This avoids back strain resulting from the practitioner reaching for supplies from the stable counter top. All supplies can be conveniently kept in a "tackle box" for easy storage and accessibility.

TABLE 6–4. *Suppliers*

1. Sclerovein
   (polidocanol—A.K.A. Aethoxysclerol)
   Vascular Products, Inc.
   35 King Street, Bristol BS.1
   402 England
   011–44–432–356437

2. Sodium tetradecyl sulfate
   (available from medical supply
   pharmacies)
   Elkins-Sinn, Inc.
   2 Esterbrook Lane
   Cherry Hill, NJ 08003–4099
   (609) 424–3700

3. 23.4% Hypertonic saline
   (available from medical supply
   pharmacies)
   Lyphomed
   Division of Fujisawn USA, Inc.
   3 Parkway North
   Deerfield, IL 60015–2548
   (800) 888–7704

4. Doppler
   Parks Medical Electronics
   P.O. Box 5669
   Aloha, OR 97007
   (503) 649–7007
   Model 811B

5. AV-1000 Light Reflection Rheography
   Hemodynamics, Inc.
   Mobile Diagnostic Services of America
   P.O. Box 610032
   Dallas, TX 75261–0032
   (817) 481–7517

6. Support hose
   Sigvaris
   P.O. Box 570
   Bradford, CT 06405
   (800) 322–7744

7. Support hose
   Medi-Strumpf, American Weco
   76 West Seegers
   Arlington Heights, IL 60005
   (800) 633–6334

8. Support hose
   The Jobst Institute, Inc.
   P.O. Box 653
   Toledo, Ohio 43694
   (800) 537–1063

9. Needles
   Acuderm, Inc.
   5370 N.W. 35th Terrace
   Ft. Lauderdale, FL 33309
   (305) 733–6935

10. Medi-Rip reorder #0520
    3" Rolls, 12 per box
    Conco Medical Company
    481 Lakeshore Parkway
    Rockhill, SC 29730
    (803) 325–7600

11. Elastikon tape reorder #5174
    2" Rolls, 6 per box
    Johnson & Johnson
    425 Hoes Lane
    PO Box 6800
    Piscataway, NJ 08855–6800
    (800) 255–2500

12. Brochure: "Treatment of Leg Veins"
    North American Society of Phlebology
    930 N. Meacham Rd.
    Schaumburg, IL 60173
    (708) 330–9830

The patient is first placed supine for injections on the anterior legs and thighs. Bending the patient's knee and rotating it medially and laterally allows easy access to the medial and lateral aspects of both thighs and legs. The patient is then turned prone for completion of the injections on the posterior aspect. This system works well to ensure that all the spider veins have been visualized and none are missed.

The lighting must be optimal. Indirect lighting has been reported to be better than direct for visualization of spider veins. A portable light or movable ceiling-mounted lights are recommended for easy focusing as the practitioner changes areas during the procedure.

The areas to be injected are wiped clean with alcohol. This serves two purposes. The alcohol acts as an antiseptic and also changes the index of refraction of the skin so that the spider veins are more visible.

Magnification also aids in visualization of the spider veins. Optimal visualization of the spider veins promotes accuracy and efficiency of injection. Ocular loupes (X2 or X3 magnification), magnifying visor or magnification ring with light are all good options. However, one of the most comfortable, easy, and inexpensive options is a pair of magnifying glasses (X2 magnification, 18–in focal length), which can be purchased in most drug stores.

The injections are performed in most cases with 30–gauge 1/2–in disposable needles. These needles are small enough to enter small-caliber spider veins that appear more minute than the needle itself. In addition, 31– or 32–gauge needles are available, but they easily clog on puncturing the skin and are nondisposable, so they are not practical. The needle is carefully bent to a 30– to 45–degree angle so that the needle is as parallel to the skin as possible when entering the spider vein. This aids in keeping the needle at the extremely superficial level where the spider veins are located. Also, the bevel of the needle is turned upward toward the practitioner so that the needle can sometimes be seen in the lumen of the spider vein.

Small syringes of 1– to 3–cc volume are used for the injections. A convenient approach is to fill 3–cc syringes with only 1.25 to 1.5 cc of the sclerosant. In this way, the plunger is closer to the hub so that the syringe can be held and the plunger pushed with the same hand, freeing the opposite hand. In the past, glass syringes were used commonly because they afforded fine control of the injection pressure in such small, fragile veins. Another subtle advantage of glass syringes is that the higher injection pressure necessary for a perivenous infiltration would be felt immediately and would alert the practitioner to the fact that the needle was not in the vein.[1] Glass syringes, however, are non-disposable and require sterilization between patients. Because of the fear of blood-borne diseases, most sclerotherapists now use plastic syringes. Precision and control of injection pressure are not compromised with the use of plastic syringes. They are disposable, and multiple syringes can be filled in advance, adding greatly to the efficiency of the procedure.

It is recommended that gloves be worn during the procedure to protect the practitioner from contact with the patient's blood. The gloves must be very form fitting, such as surgical gloves, to decrease as much as possible the interference with palpation caused by the glove.

Maximal stability of the syringe and needle is necessary to ensure accuracy of injection. The syringe can easily be held in the dominant hand with the index and middle fingers while the thumb operates the plunger. The fifth finger rests on the patient to provide stability and retraction (Fig. 6–1). The opposite, nondominant hand is used for retraction to spread out the skin. Retraction of the skin is necessary to puncture the skin properly. An assistant is not necessary for retraction if the practitioner positions the hands properly for the injections in the manner just described.

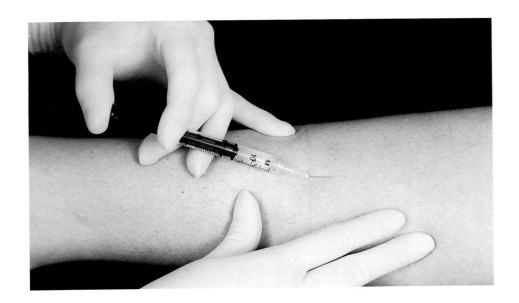

FIGURE 6–1. *Proper position of hands, syringe, and needle for injection with optimal retraction, syringe half-full, needle bent, and bevel upward.*

The site of entry into the spider vein is determined at the highest point of reflux. With the needle bent to 45 degrees and kept as parallel to the skin as possible and bevel upward, the skin is punctured approximately 1 mm from the desired location of entry into the spider vein. The bevel is then guided precisely into the spider vein, and a gentle, but bold puncture is usually necessary to enter into the vein. Sometimes a subtle "pop" can be felt as the spider vein is entered. These veins are so superficial that the needle can sometimes be seen within the vein. It is not necessary or productive to obtain a blood return from such a small lumen through such a small needle. Drawing back on the plunger in an attempt to obtain a blood return may jeopardize your precise needle placement in the lumen.

The injection is performed gently with only slight pressure on the plunger. If the needle is positioned properly in the lumen of the vein, the vein will be cleared of blood as the sclerosant is injected. This will appear as blanching of the area. In the case of an interconnected, arborizing pattern of spider veins, this blanching can be quite dramatic (Fig. 6–2). It is recommended to stop the injection of that particular site once an area of 1 to 2 cm is emptied of blood. Continuing the injection beyond this point is felt to increase the likelihood of extravasation and telangiectatic matting.[2] Telangiectatic matting appears as very fine-caliber (<0.2 mm), red spider veins which can develop as a postsclerotherapy complication around the areas injected. High injection pressures have been implicated as one of the causes of telangiectatic matting. Injections are limited to 0.5 cc of the sclerosant at any one site for the same reasons.

Some authors advocate an "air block" technique of injection.[1,3] A minute amount of air is drawn into the syringe with the needle up prior to puncturing the skin. On entering the spider vein, the air is first injected, clearing the vein and ensuring proper positioning in the lumen prior to injecting. This technique was advocated particularly with the use of hypertonic saline as the sclerosant.[3] Hypertonic saline hemolyzes red blood cells, and hemolysis causes the formation of hemosiderin. Hemosiderin deposits cause brown staining. Consequently, it was felt that evacuating the vein of blood by first injecting air

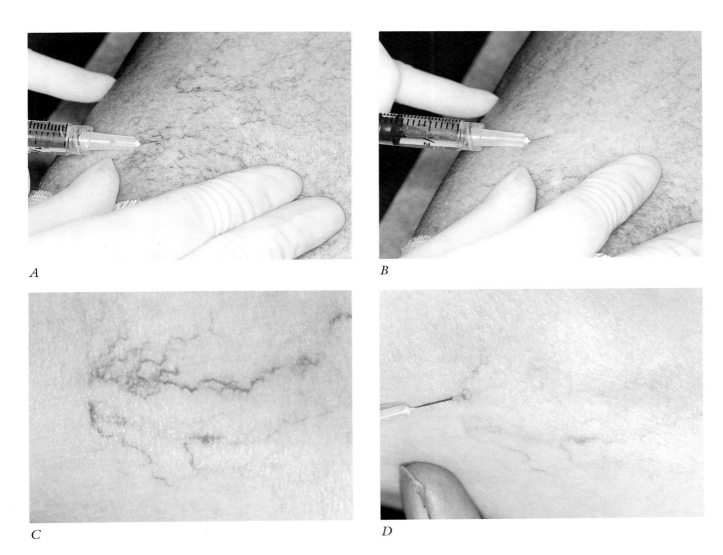

A

B

C

D

FIGURE 6–2. *A,B. Blanching is seen as the sclerosant is injected and the vein is cleared of blood. C,D. It is recommended to stop the injection after 1 to 2 cm of blanching to avoid extravasation and telangiectatic matting. Select a second injection site for the remainder of the injection.*

would prevent hemolysis and possibly any brown staining. However, the injection of air has not eliminated hemosiderin deposits and is not universally felt to be necessary even when using hypertonic saline.[4]

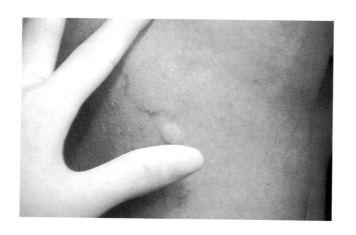

FIGURE 6–3. *A skin wheal indicative of perivascular infiltration. Immediately abort the injection. Then digitally compress the injection site to diffuse the sclerosant so as to prevent skin necrosis.*

In the event the lumen is missed, a wheal will be raised at the injection site as the sclerosant is injected. Perivascular infiltration of most sclerosants can result in skin necrosis (Fig. 6–3).

At the first hint of an extravasation, abort the injection at that site and digitally compress the injection site. This will dilute the extravasated sclerosant by diffusion and hopefully avert significant injury to the skin. In the case of an inadvertent extravasation, the site also can be injected with normal saline or a local anesthetic to further dilute the sclerosant and decrease the pain that accompanies extravasation of some of the sclerosants. It is prudent to keep handy during the procedure a syringe filled with normal saline or local anesthetic in the case of extravasation. It is recommended to utilize a different syringe size for this, such as a TB syringe, to avoid confusion with the syringes containing the sclerosant.

Since the spider veins are so superficial in most cases of missing the lumen, the needle is deep to the vein. Maintaining digital pressure on this failed site, select a second injection site into the spider vein, making sure that the needle is properly bent and is as parallel to the skin as possible to ensure that the needle stays superficial as you advance into the vein.

Occasionally, a different method of injection may be used in cases of larger reticular veins (Fig. 6–4). These veins have been mapped out

SCLEROTHERAPY OF SPIDER VEINS

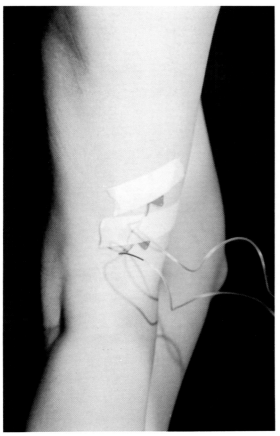

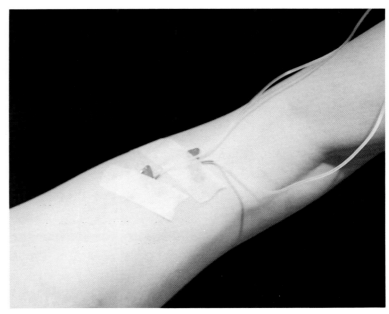

A   B

previously and are again confirmed in location with the patient standing. The injection sites are marked at the point of maximum reflux and
at 5–cm intervals along the reticular vein. The patient is placed supine
or sitting with the leg hanging over the side of the table, or standing
if the vein is not visible supine. The same venipuncture technique is
used on the reticular vein as on the smaller spider veins, except a larger
25–gauge butterfly needle is used on the reticular vein. After entering
the lumen, the position of the needle is confirmed by aspirating blood
in the butterfly tubing, which is then reinjected to prevent clogging.
The needle is then taped in position with paper tape. This is repeated at
each injection site along the vein path as marked. The patient is then
placed supine and the leg elevated to 30 degrees to empty the vein of
blood. This allows better contact of the sclerosant with the vein wall
and prevents dilution of the sclerosant. The position of the needle in

FIGURE 6–4. *A.*
Injection method for reticular
veins using 25–gauge butterfly
needles at 5–cm intervals. The
needle is inserted in the vein
with the leg dependent, and the
needle position is confirmed by
aspirating blood. B. The needle
is taped in place, and the leg is
elevated to empty the vein
before injecting 0.5 cc of
sclerosant at each site.

the vein lumen is again confirmed by aspirating blood in the tubing, and 0.5 cc of sclerosant is injected at each site. If possible, the 5–cm segment of vein around the needle can be compressed with the index and ring fingers as the sclerosant is injected to maximize the contact between the sclerosant and the vein wall in that isolated segment. The middle finger can be placed over the needle entry site to detect any extravasation as the sclerosant is injected. This injection technique for large reticular veins is adopted from that commonly used for varicose veins.[5]

COMPRESSION DEBATE

After the injection is complete in a specific area, compression is applied. As the compression is applied, a hyperemic reaction in the sclerosed spider vein may be apparent, and this is the expected reaction to the sclerosant (Fig. 6–5). A cotton ball over the injection site covered with elastic tape will suffice in most cases of spider veins. The value of additional compression in the form of compression bandages or stockings is uncertain in the case of spider veins. However, following sclerotherapy of varicose veins, compression for 6 weeks has been strongly advocated by the pioneers of sclerotherapy in England and Ireland.[6,7]

One study measured the pressure exerted by compression bandages over time and found a fall in pressure to zero at only 6 to 8 hours.[8] This raised the question of the actual value of compression after only this very short time. Several studies have been conducted for the purpose of determining the optimal length of compression time after sclerotherapy. Various studies have found no difference in results between 3 weeks, 3 days, or 8 hours versus 6 weeks of compression.[9–11] The French phlebologists in general use compression after sclerotherapy in a more limited role than the Irish and British schools.[12]

The pressing question after sclerotherapy of spider veins is the need for graduated compression at all, even for a brief length of time. Unlike the varicose vein patient, the patient with cosmetic spider veins has little tolerance for expensive, uncomfortable, and inconvenient post-

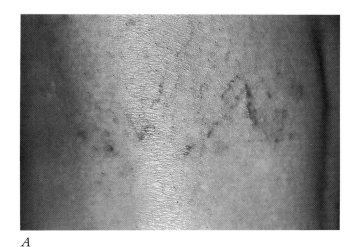

A

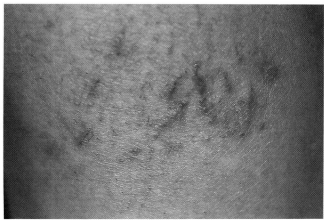

B

FIGURE 6–5.
A. *Before sclerotherapy.*
B. *Approximately 30 seconds after sclerotherapy. Notice the intense hyperemic reaction that develops in the spider vein.*

sclerotherapy protocols. This is true no matter how badly the appearance of the spider veins bothers the patient. Unfortunately, the area of the country where people are most bothered by the appearance of their spider veins is the Sun Belt area, where shorts are worn year-round, and this is where compressive bandages can be unbearably hot and uncomfortable. In addition to being uncomfortable, compression can be dangerous.[13]

According to a preliminary report on the use of compression after sclerotherapy of leg telangiectasias less than 1 mm in diameter, greater resolution was achieved using 30 to 40 mmHg of graduated compression for 72 hours when the telangiectasias were located on the distal leg or were greater than 0.5 mm in diameter.[14] There also was a decrease in postsclerotherapy hyperpigmentation from 40.5 to 28.5 percent. Higher pressures over the sclerosing site have been advocated using foam pads or two stockings to completely empty the superficial veins of blood.[14,15]

Goldman points out the five purposes of postsclerotherapy compression.[16] Opposition of the vein walls can enhance fibrosis and decrease thrombus formation (thereby decreasing the risk of postsclerotherapy hyperpigmentation, recanalization, or telangiectatic matting). Compression decreases superficial venous pressure in patients with venous insufficiency and improves the function of the venous calf pump.[17,18]

In light of these theoretical considerations, as well as the controversy regarding the value and timing of postsclerotherapy compression, a practical approach is in order for patients with spider veins. In patients with smaller spider veins, a cotton ball fixed by elastic tape will most likely suffice. In patients with larger spider veins, especially distally, wrapping the legs with a compressive bandage for a few days is indicated. Patients who have developed postsclerotherapy thrombi or hyperpigmentation in the past should be treated with 30 to 40 mmHg of graduated compression for 72 hours after sclerotherapy to decrease the likelihood of these adverse sequelae. These patients are also more accepting of the additional cost and inconvenience if it may hasten their ultimate recovery and improve their result (Fig. 6–6).

Another practical alternative to cotton balls and tape alone in patients with spider veins is the addition of over-the-counter support panty-hose. These exact a pressure of 15 to 20 mmHg, are inexpensive, and serve to hold the tapes on. Because this compression is nongraduated, one study finds these over-the-counter support hose to be detrimental to venous return.[19] The issue of whether this additional local compression is so beneficial that it outweighs this concern is still debatable.[20] One compromise is the *sheer* graduated support pantyhose now available from Jobst for approximately $18.50.

POSTPROCEDURE CARE

Following sclerotherapy, the patient is given a printed instruction sheet with explicit directions on posttreatment care (Table 6–5). The patient is encouraged to ambulate in order to decrease the risk of deep vein thrombosis. Patients are reminded to avoid activities that increase venous pressure in the legs, such as prolonged sitting or standing, "pounding-type" exercises such as high-impact aerobics or running, heavy weight-lifting, or squatting. They are asked to remove the tapes from their legs in 48 hours following the procedure. This is an arbitrary

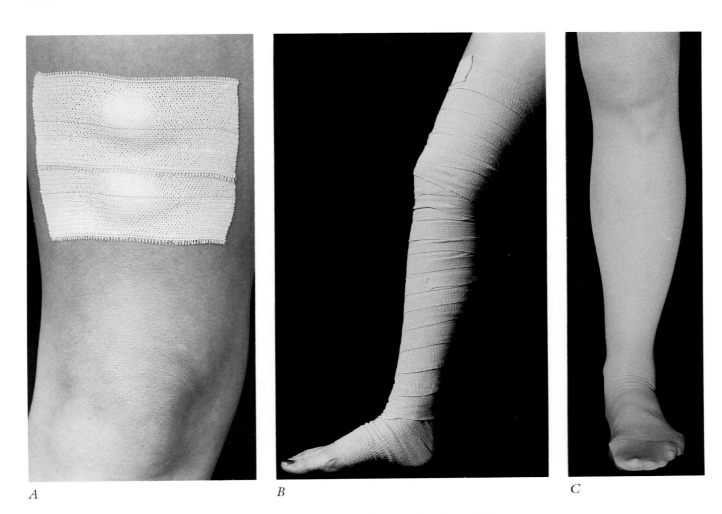

A　　　　　　　　　　　　　*B*　　　　　　　　　　　　　*C*

F I G U R E 6–6. *Three methods of compression after sclerotherapy. A. Cotton balls with tape are the most common method of compression after sclerotherapy of spider veins. These may be reinforced with over-the-counter pantyhose. B. The legs may be wrapped with a compression bandage over the cotton balls and tape in patients with larger or extensive spider veins. C. Graduated compression stockings (30 to 40 mmHg) may be advisable, particularly in patients who have developed hyperpigmentation after sclerotherapy in the past.*

time chosen to allow partial resolution of the initial hyperemic reaction and irritation from the needle puncture and so minimize patient concern. The patient is again reminded to expect some bruising that should gradually improve with time.

TABLE 6–5. *Spider Vein Injections Post-treatment Care*

1. Walking is encouraged after the injections.
2. Avoid prolonged sitting and standing, pounding-type exercises, squatting, and heavy weight-lifting after the injections.
3. Remove tapes in 48 hours.
4. If your legs were wrapped after the injections, remove the wrapping in 48 hours. If the wrapping feels "too tight" or if you experience numbness or discoloration of your toes, call the office and loosen the wraps.
5. Wear support hose when up as much as possible and bring a pair to each treatment session.
6. If special stockings were ordered and placed on your legs after the injections, wear them when up for 72 hours. You may remove them to sleep, but only with your legs up in bed and you must reapply them in the morning before you hang your legs out of bed.

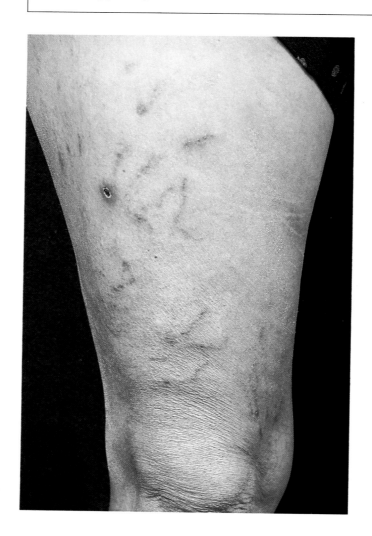

FIGURE 6–7.
Cutaneous necrosis after sclerotherapy surrounded by extensive thrombi in injected telangiectasias. These thrombi should be evacuated to decrease hyperpigmentation.

FOLLOW-UP INJECTION SCHEDULE

An appointment is made for follow-up approximately 1 week after the first treatment session. By this time, the initial bruising has started to subside. Any area of impending necrosis will have started to demarcate. Any superficial thrombi will have liquefied and should be evacuated. (Fig. 6–7).

If any small scabs or blisters are present at the injection site, the patient should be advised to wash this area twice a day to decrease contamination and reduce the risk of infection. Also, the areas of eschar should be protected from the sun. Careful technique and low concentrations of weak sclerosing agents for the sclerotherapy of spider veins should minimize the risk of development of cutaneous necrosis. If a small scab does develop, however, it usually will heal in 6 weeks. The resulting scar after healing by secondary intention is smaller than the original involved area secondary to contraction. The scar usually remains pink for approximately 6 months as the scar matures. This gradually fades, resulting in a small hypo- or hyperpigmented area. The patient should protect the scar from tanning during this maturation phase in order to decrease the incidence of hyperpigmentation of the scar.

The treatment sessions are scheduled approximately at monthly intervals until the treatment plan is completed. In a month's time the sclerosis achieved at each session should be evident and the bruising resolved. If the patient has an extensive number of spider veins so that only one area or leg can be sclerosed at each session, treatments can be scheduled as frequently as weekly on different areas.

REFERENCES

1. Sigg K. Treatment of varicose veins by injection sclerotherapy: A method practised in Switzerland. In Hobbs JT, ed: The Treatment of Venous Disorders. Philadelphia: Lippincott, 1977, p 118.
2. Ouvry PA. Telangiectasia and sclerotherapy. J Dermatol Surg Oncol 1989; 15:177–181.
3. Foley WT. The eradication of venous blemishes. Cutis 1975; 15:665–668.

4. Alderman DB. Therapy for essential cutaneous telangiectasias. Postgrad Med 1977; 61:91–95.

5. Fegan WG. Treatment of varicose veins by injection-compression: A method practiced in Eire. In Hobbs JT, ed: The Treatment of Venous Disorders. Philadelphia: Lippincott, 1977, pp 109–110.

6. Fegan WG. Treatment of varicose veins by injection-compression: A method practised in Eire. In Hobbs JT, ed: The Treatment of Venous Disorders. Philadelphia: Lippincott, 1977, pp 109–112.

7. Hobbs JT. A random trial of the treatment of varicose veins by surgery and sclerotherapy. In Hobbs JT, ed: The Treatment of Venous Disorders. Philadelphia: Lippincott, 1977, p 201.

8. Raj TB, Goddard M, Makin GS. How long do compression bandages maintain their pressure during ambulatory treatment of varicose veins? Br J Surg 1980; 67:122–124.

9. Batch AJG, Wickremesinghe SS, Gannon ME, et al. Randomised trial of bandaging after sclerotherapy for varicose veins. Br Med J 1980; 281:423.

10. Fraser IA, Perry EP, Hatton M, Watkin DFL. Prolonged bandaging is not required following sclerotherapy of varicose veins. Br J Surg 1985; 72:488–490.

11. Raj TB, Makin GS. A random, controlled trial of two forms of compression bandaging in outpatient sclerotherapy of varicose veins. J Surg Res 1981; 31:440–445.

12. Wallois P. The conditions necessary to achieve an effective sclerosant treatment. Phlebologie 1982; 35:337–348.

13. Callam MJ, Ruckley CV, Dale JJ, et al. Hazards of compression treatment of the leg: An estimate from Scottish surgeons. Br Med J 1987; 295:1382.

14. Goldman MP, Beaudoing D, Marley W, et al. Compression in the treatment of leg telangiectasia: A preliminary report. J Dermatol Surg Oncol 1990; 16:322–325.

15. Fentem PH, Goddard M, Gooden BA, et al. Control of distension of varicose veins achieved by leg bandages, as used after injection sclerotherapy. Br Med J 1976; 2:725–727.

16. Goldman MP. Compression in the treatment of leg telangiectasia: Theoretical considerations. J Dermatol Surg Oncol 1989; 15:184–188.

17. Somerville JJF, Brow GO, Byrne PJ, et al. The effect of elastic stockings on superficial venous pressures in patients with venous insufficiency. Br J Surg 1974; 61:979–981.

18. Struckmann J. Compression stockings and their effect on the venous pump: A comparative study. Phlebology 1986; 1:37–45.

19. Godin MS, Rice JC, Kerstein MD. Effect of commercially available pantyhose on venous return in the lower extremity. J Vasc Surg 1987; 5:844–848.

20. de Groot WP. Practical phlebology: Sclerotherapy of large veins. J Dermatol Surg Oncol 1991; 17:589–595.

ADDITIONAL READINGS

Biegeleisen HI. Telangiectasia associated with varicose veins: Treatment by a micro-injection technique. JAMA 1934; 102:2092–2094.

Bodian E. Sclerotherapy. Dialogues Dermatol 1983; 13:(tape)1.

Bodian EL. Techniques of sclerotherapy for sunburst venous blemishes. J Dermatol Surg Oncol 1985; 11:696–704.

Bodian EL. Sclerotherapy. Semin Dermatol 1987; 6:238–248.

Goldman MP, Bennett RG. Treatment of telangiectasia: A review. J Am Acad Dermatol 1987; 17:167–182.

Goldman PM. Sclerotherapy for superficial venules and telangiectasias of the lower extremities. Dermatol Clin 1987; 5:369–379.

Green D. Compression sclerotherapy techniques. Dermatol Clin 1989; 7:137–146.

Johnson G Jr, Kupper C, Farrar DJ, Swallow RT. Graded compression stockings. Custom vs noncustom. Arch Surg 1982; 117:69–72.

Ouvry PA, Davy A. The sclerotherapy of telangiectasia. Phlébologie 1982; 35:349–359.

Partsch H. Compression therapy of the legs A review. J Dermatol Surg Oncol 1991; 17: 799–805.

Pierce HE. Management of unsightly micro-varicosities. Am J Cosmetic Surg 1984; 1: 45–47.

Shields JL, Jansen GT. Therapy for superficial telangiectasias of the lower extremities. J Dermatol Surg Oncol 1982; 8:857–860.

7

RESULTS OF SCLEROTHERAPY

PATIENT SATISFACTION

The key to patient satisfaction is adequate pretreatment counseling. It is important to prepare patients for the fact that the legs will look worse before they look better. Patients should expect some bruising at the injection sites that may take up to a month to resolve completely. As the bruises resolve, patients will notice gradual lightening of the spider veins after each treatment session. A reasonable amount of lightening of the spider veins that can be expected after each treatment session is 50 to 60 percent (Fig. 7–1). If the expected lightening is not achieved, then, on occasion, a change of the sclerosing agent may be necessary. The patient is more tolerant of this change if warned of the possibility before scheduling the treatment sessions.

A treatment plan including the approximate number of treatment sessions must be formulated and discussed with the patient prior to scheduling. The patient also needs to be informed of the approximate length of time needed to complete the treatment plan, as well as the cost of each treatment session. This allows the patient to budget the time and money necessary to achieve the desired result. The patient must be advised that the treatment plan is not absolute and may require revision depending on the patient's individual response to treatment. The patient must understand that any of the complications may require further expense and recovery time. All these points must be addressed in the pretreatment counseling to avoid patient dissatisfaction. A checklist

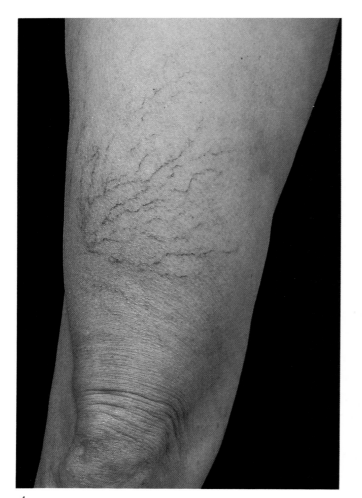

A

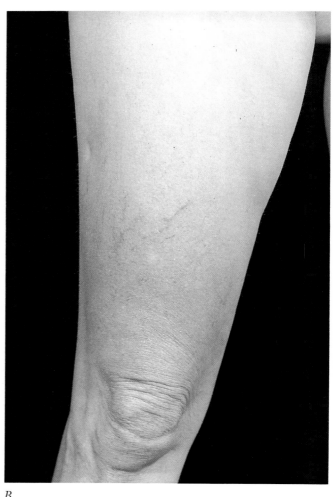

B

FIGURE 7–1. A. Before
sclerotherapy. B. Six weeks after
one sclerotherapy treatment
with 0.5% polidocanol showing
degree of lightening that can be
expected after a single
injection. Additional
injections at approximately
monthly intervals are necessary
for further obliteration.

of these points (Table 7–1) is reviewed and signed by the patient prior
to scheduling and is placed in the permanent record.

Most patients find the discomfort and inconvenience of the treatment
minimal and the rewards great. The agony women feel over the appearance of these spider veins should not be underestimated. Women are
extremely self-conscious about them because of their high visibility.
Many women limit their wardrobe to long pants and skirts to hide their
legs because of the spider veins. Women complain bitterly about them.
Unfortunately, their cry for help many times falls on deaf ears. A recent
poll of gynecologists in one medical community confirmed the negative perception that the general medical community has about sclerotherapy, leaving women frustrated in their search for treatment.

SCLEROTHERAPY OF SPIDER VEINS

T A B L E 7–1. *Spider Vein Checklist*

Name:_____

Physician: _____

Date:_____

1. _____ Sclerotherapy involves injection of a medication in the spider veins to "close" them off from filling so they are less visible.

2. _____ We will never be able to obliterate every spider vein but will try to decrease the venous appearance of your legs with gradual lightening of the spider veins with each session.

3. _____ Your legs will look worse initially after the injections with bruising which lasts up to a month.

4. _____ You will have tapes on your legs for 48 hours after the injections.

5. _____ Your treatment will take several sessions and we can only estimate for you the number that will be required.

6. _____ The treatment sessions are usually scheduled at monthly intervals on the same areas but the time intervals can vary.

7. _____ You should wear your support hose continuously for 72 hours after the injections and then as much as possible. You may remove them at night but replace them before putting your legs down in the morning.

8. _____ Bring your support hose to each treatment session.

9. _____ Do not put creams on your legs on the treatment day.

10. _____ You are encouraged to walk after the injections.

11. _____ You should avoid prolonged sitting and standing, pounding types of exercise, squatting, and heavy weight lifting after the injections.

12. _____ You may have some cramping in your legs for a few days after the injections.

13. _____ You will feel small needle sticks and possibly mild burning upon injection but this pain is usually minimal.

14. _____ The spider veins can recur, and you may require touch-up injections in the future.

15. _____ Possible complications of sclerotherapy include hyperpigmentation (brown discoloration), scarring, telangiectatic matting (appearance of fine red spiders), allergic reactions, thrombophlebitis (inflammation of veins), and deep vein thrombosis (clots in deep veins).

16. _____ Complications can require medical treatment, more expense, and greater recovery time.

17. _____ You can develop small superficial clots that may need to be evacuated usually at approximately one week after the injections.

Name:_____

Physician:_____

Certification of Informed Consent

SPIDER VEIN INJECTIONS

Information listed on this spider vein injection sheet has been thoroughly explained to me. I have been able to ask questions and am satisfied that I understand the procedure and its risks and benefits. The general information sheet on spider vein injections has been given to me.

_____
Signed

_____
Dated

Hopefully, as the medical con
patient satisfaction with scle
change so that patients will b
deserve.[1]

PERMANENCE O

Recurrence of the original spider veins after treatment is due to re-canalization of the vein lumen. The larger the amount of thrombus formation in the vein lumen following sclerotherapy, the greater is the likelihood of recanalization. Every effort must be made to minimize thrombus formation with the appropriate choice of sclerosant and concentration, as well as postsclerotherapy compression. If thrombus is apparent after sclerotherapy, evacuation of the thrombus is indicated and may enhance the permanence of the result.

In general, the same sclerosed vessels do not reappear with time, although one author has noted the recurrence of telangiectasias in a lighter form in 1 to 5 years.[2] The treatment obviously is limited only to those spider veins evident at a certain point in time. Since the etiology of spider veins is multifactorial, the development of new spider veins with time is not completely preventable.[3] It is not possible to predict the probability of progression of venous insufficiency in each individual. Certainly reevaluation of the venous system may be necessary in the future to assess the continued suitability of the patient for sclerotherapy.

The majority of the spider vein patients are satisfied with the results of the sclerotherapy. They occasionally return every few years for "touch-up" injections of new spider veins that have developed in the interim.

REALISTIC EXPECTATIONS

Realistic expectations are the key to patient satisfaction. The goal of sclerotherapy is to decrease the objectionable venous appearance of the

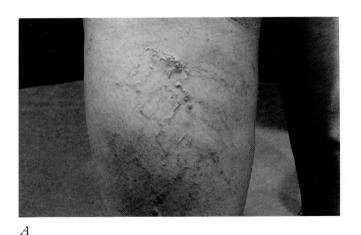

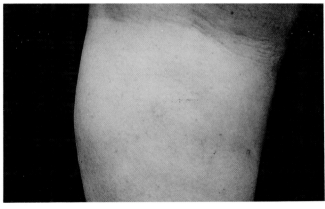

A

B

FIGURE 7–2. *A. Before sclerotherapy. B. Two and a half years after sclerotherapy with 0.5% sodium tetradecyl sulfate in three treatment sessions.*

legs (Figs. 7–2 to 7–5). Complete obliteration of every telangiectasia is unrealistic and should not be promised. The aesthetic limitations must be addressed prior to scheduling the procedure.

The practitioner also must be honest in deciding when the limits of sclerotherapy have been reached. Continuing the treatment beyond this point results in a disproportionately high risk for the benefit achieved. Some patients, unfortunately, will point to telangiectasias that can barely be seen even with magnification. At this point, the patient can be encouraged to "wait and see" if any develop to significant size for sclerotherapy to be feasible. A referral for an alternate method of treatment such as laser therapy also may be suggested at this point.

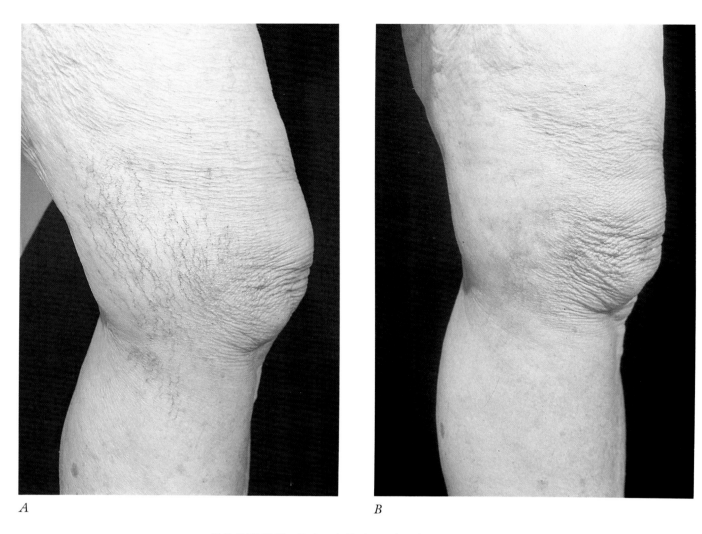

A

B

FIGURE 7–3. *A. Before sclerotherapy. B. One and a half years after sclerotherapy with 18.7% hypertonic saline plus 0.4% lidocaine (Xylocaine) in two treatment sessions.*

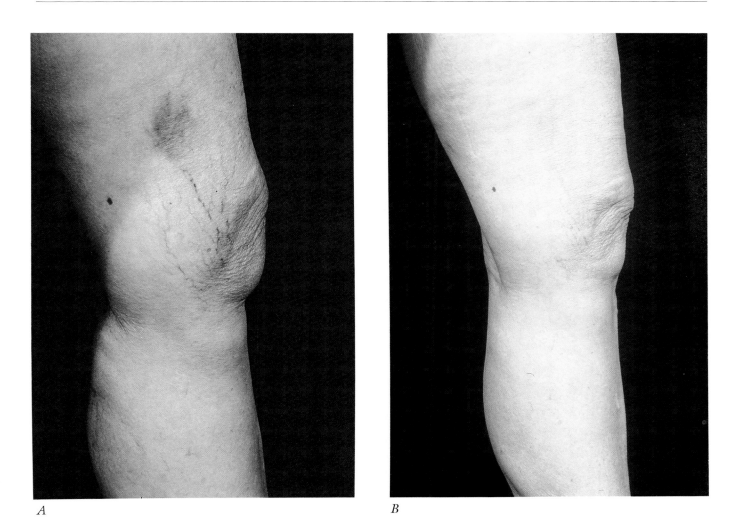

A   *B*

FIGURE 7–4. *A. Before sclerotherapy. B. Six months after sclerotherapy with 0.75% polidocanol in two treatment sessions.*

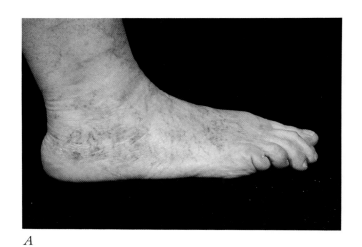

A

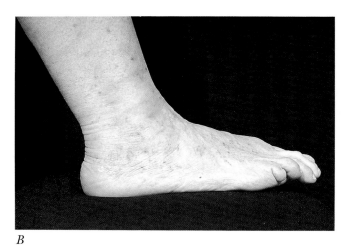

B

FIGURE 7–5. *A. Before sclerotherapy. B. Two years after sclerotherapy with 0.33% sodium tetradecyl sulfate in three treatment sessions.*

REFERENCES

1. Weiss RA, Weiss MA, Goldman MP. Physician's negative perception of sclerotherapy for venous disorders: Review of a 7–year positive experience with modern sclerotherapy. South Med J 1992; 85:1101–1106.

2. Alderman DB. Therapy for essential cutaneous telangiectasias. Postgrad Med 1977; 61:91–95.

3. Sadick NS. Predisposing factors of varicose and telangiectatic leg veins. J Dermatol Surg Oncol 1992; 18:883–886.

ADDITIONAL READINGS

Carlin MC, Ratz JL. Treatment of telangiectasia: Comparison of sclerosing agents. J Dermatol Surg Oncol 1987; 13:1181–1184.

Duffy DM. Small vessel sclerotherapy: An overview. In Callen JP, Dahl MV, Golitz LE, et al, eds: Advances in Dermatology. Vol 3. Chicago: Year Book Medical, 1988, pp 221–242.

Duffy DM. Sclerotherapy: A debate on various issues (letter). J Dermatol Surg Oncol 1991; 17:625.

Goldman MP. The role of the American dermatologist in phlebology (editorial). J Dermatol Surg Oncol 1989; 15:135.

Goldman MP, Bennett RG. Treatment of telangiectasia: A review. J Am Acad Dermatol 1987; 17:167–182.

Goldman PM. Sclerotherapy for superficial venules and telangiectasias of the lower extremities. Dermatol Clin 1987; 5:369–379.

Green D. Compression sclerotherapy techniques. Dermatol Clin 1989; 7:137–146.

Ouvry PA. Telangiectasia and sclerotherapy. J Dermatol Surg Oncol 1989; 15:177–181.

Puissegur-Lupo ML. Sclerotherapy: Review of results and complications in 200 patients. J Dermatol Surg Oncol 1989; 15:214–219.

Schmier AA. Clinical comparison of sclerosing solutions in injection treatment of varicose veins. Am J Surg 1937; 36:389–397.

Weiss RA, Weiss MA. Sclerotherapy. In Wheeland RG, ed: Cutaneous Surgery. Philadelphia: Saunders, 1994, pp 951–981.

COMPLICATIONS OF SCLEROTHERAPY

SCLEROTHERAPY of spider veins is not a perfect procedure. Adverse sequelae are not uncommon but usually are relatively minor and self-limiting. A minor complication usually results in an aesthetic imperfection that is nominal compared with the aesthetic improvement achieved by eradication of the spider veins. Consequently, a minor complication, although causing great patient concern initially, becomes well tolerated as the adverse sequela fades with time. These possible complications include pigment changes, cutaneous necrosis, telangiectatic matting, allergic reaction to the medication, superficial thrombi and thrombophlebitis, and deep vein thrombosis.

HYPERPIGMENTATION

Hyperpigmentation is the most common adverse sequela following sclerotherapy. It is also the cause of great patient concern because, in severe cases, it can replace the purple vein path with a brown, linear streak (Fig. 8–1). This streak is caused by hemosiderin deposits rather than melanin, as confirmed by histologic examination of biopsies of postsclerotherapy hyperpigmentation.[1] The hemosiderin deposition occurs as a result of extravasation of red blood cells through the ruptured vein wall into the dermis. Injury to the vein wall can be minimized by proper technique, low injection pressures, and the selection

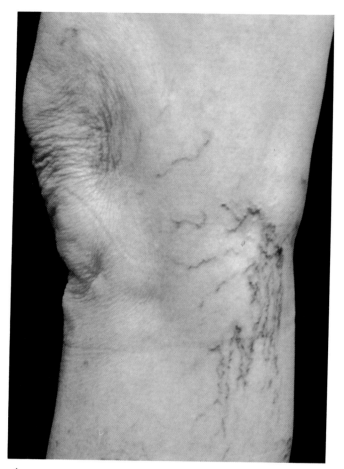

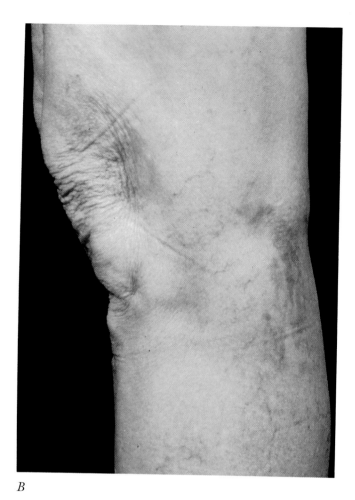

A

B

F I G U R E 8–1.
A. Before sclerotherapy. B. Hyperpigmentation 2 months after sclerotherapy secondary to hemosiderin deposit.

of appropriately weak sclerosants in low concentrations for use in spider veins. Of the most popular sclerosants used for spider veins, the incidence of postsclerotherapy hyperpigmentation varies from 5 to 33 percent for sodium tetradecal sulfate, 10.9 to 33 percent for hypertonic saline, and 10.7 to 30.7 percent for polidocanol.[2–6] Other authors have noted hyperpigmentation to occur more frequently with sodium tetradecal sulfate than with hypertonic saline or polidocanol, and the pigment has been noted to persist longer following injection with sodium tetradecal sulfate.[7–9] Decreasing the concentration of sodium tetradechol for sclerotherapy of spider veins from 1% to 0.33% resulted in a decrease in the hyperpigmentation rate from 33 to 5 percent.[2] Certainly the concentration of the sclerosing agent should be limited to that necessary to cause fibrosis of the vessel without excessive damage in order to minimize the risk of hyperpigmentation, as well as other complications of sclerotherapy.

The hyperpigmentation has been postulated to be a result of thrombus formation.[10] Consequently, measures that limit thrombus formation decrease the risk and amount of hyperpigmentation.[11] Compression may decrease thrombus formation by opposing the vessel walls.[12] For this reason, it is prudent to use maximal compression, such as 30– to 40–mmHg graduated compressive stockings for 72 hours after sclerotherapy in patients who have experienced postsclerotherapy hyperpigmentation in the past.

When thrombi are seen in the lumen of spider veins after sclerotherapy, removal with a 25–gauge needle, a lancet, or a no. 11 blade minimizes the risk of hyperpigmentation[10] (Fig. 8–2). The coagulum liquefies at approximately 1 week after the injections, making the evacuation possible at this time. If the thrombi are extensive, this may require several office visits, since patients can only tolerate the discomfort associated with clot evacuation for a brief time.

FIGURE 8–2. *A. Removal of thrombi in the lumen of a spider vein with a 25–gauge needle 1 week after sclerotherapy. B. The liquefied coagulum being expressed. C. Typical appearance of removed clot. A few other thrombi still require declotting.*

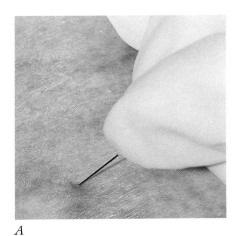
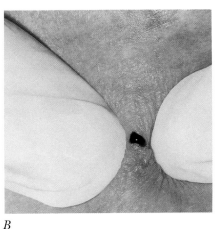
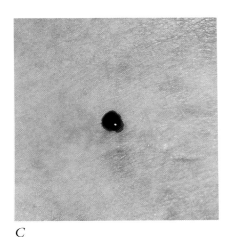

A   *B*   *C*

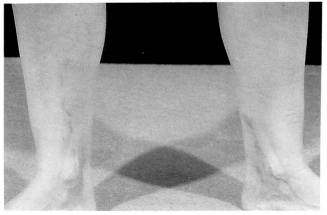

A

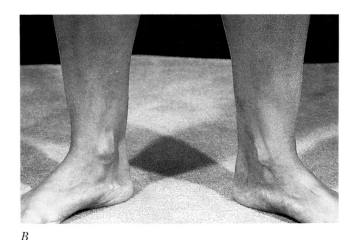

B

FIGURE 8–3. *A. Hyperpigmentation of medial legs and ankles 2 months after sclerotherapy. B. Two years later, the hyperpigmentation has lightened so much it is barely visible.*

Once hyperpigmentation is established, it definitely fades with time. A substantial lightening usually occurs over the first 6 months; however, a gradual lightening process continues over 24 months[1,8,13] (Fig. 8–3).

Various modalities have been used to remove the hyperpigmentation, including bleaching agents (trichloroacetic acid and hydroquinone), cryotherapy (liquid nitrogen or solid CO_2), and the laser (copper vapor and pulsed-dye lasers). Since the bleaching agents are only effective on melanin rather than hemosiderin, they are not effective in treating postsclerotherapy hyperpigmentation. Cryotherapy also has had questionable success.[8,14] More recently, the copper vapor and pulsed-dye lasers have shown promise in treating refractory postsclerotherapy hyperpigmentation in limited numbers of patients, with 69 percent significant clearing of the pigmentation with use of the copper vapor laser and 27 percent with the pulsed-dye laser.[15,16]

CUTANEOUS NECROSIS

Cutaneous necrosis is uncommon after sclerotherapy of spider veins; however, it can occur even if an appropriate sclerosant in a weak concentration is used. It can be produced by inadvertent infiltration of the sclerosant in the perivascular tissue or by inadvertent injection into an arteriovenous anastomosis.[17]

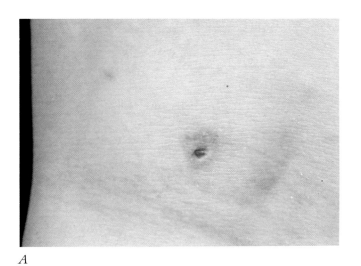
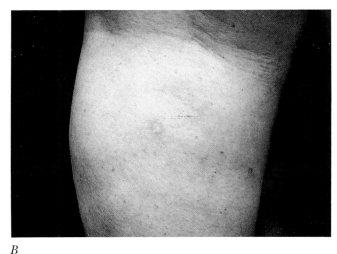

A   B

FIGURE 8–4. *A. Small area of skin necrosis 2 weeks after sclerotherapy.
B. Small hypopigmented scar with hyperpigmentation around periphery
2½ years after sclerotherapy.*

The weaker the sclerosing agent and solution, the less is the risk of ulceration. Sodium tetradecal sulfate is more toxic than hypertonic saline, which is more toxic than polidocanol.[7,8,14,18] Polidocanol is so mild that in concentrations of 0.25% to 0.5%, deliberate perivascular injection has been used to eradicate very fine telangiectasias that could not be injected intravascularly.[19] However, even polidocanol in higher concentrations can produce slough, although rarely. As with all sclerosing agents, the less concentrated the solution, the less is the possibility of skin slough. For this reason, it has been suggested that the concentration of sodium tetradecal sulfate be limited to 0.33% for sclerotherapy of spider veins.[14] The objective is to minimize the risk with use of the least toxic sclerosing agent in the least concentration that will effectively obliterate the spider veins in each individual case.

If an ulceration does occur, it is usually small (5 to 7 mm) if an appropriate sclerosant and solution for spider veins was used for the injections. By 1 to 2 weeks postinjection, the area will develop a small, dry eschar with a narrow border of erythema surrounding it (Fig. 8–4). The patient should be instructed to wash the area daily to avoid infection. The ulceration heals by secondary intention usually within 6 weeks. This leaves a small vaccination mark-like scar following a scar maturation period of approximately 6 months. The scar is usually slightly hypopigmented compared with the surrounding skin and is fairly inconspicuous. Sun exposure should be avoided during the scar maturation phase to prevent hyperpigmentation of the scar.

TELANGIECTATIC MATTING

Telangiectatic matting is defined as a network of very fine red telangiectasias, less than 0.2 mm in diameter, that can occur surrounding the area of a previously sclerosed spider vein (Fig. 8–5). The etiology of telangiectatic matting is uncertain. It may be related to perivascular inflammation that occurs following excessive injury to the vein wall leading to extravasation of red blood cells.[20] Various factors have been implicated as possible causes of telangiectatic matting following sclerotherapy of spider veins. These include the use of stronger sclerosants, high concentrations of sclerosants, inadequate compression, and high injection pressures.

The incidence of postsclerotherapy telangiectatic matting has been estimated at approximately 5 percent.[2,8] The incidence of telangiectatic matting can be affected by both the type of sclerosant and the concentration. In one study comparing the incidence of telangiectatic matting

FIGURE 8–5.
Telangiectatic matting in the vicinity of a previously sclerosed spider vein.

after sclerotherapy with 23% hypertonic saline versus 1% polidocanol, the incidence of telangiectatic matting at 1 month was 13 percent for the hypertonic saline group and 33 percent for the polidocanol group. At 6 months, the incidence decreased to 2 percent for the hypertonic saline group and 9 percent for the polidocanol group. When the concentration of polidocanol was decreased from 1% to 0.5%, the patients then demonstrated no telangiectatic matting.[5]

A higher incidence of telangiectatic matting is felt to occur following excessive thrombus formation. Telangiectasias are noted to appear during the reabsorption of the thrombi.[21] The use of compression after sclerotherapy, by minimizing the amount of thrombosis, may decrease the incidence of telangiectatic matting.[22]

High injection pressures and a large volume of sclerosant at each injection point, resulting in a large area of blanching, are other factors implicated in a higher incidence of postsclerotherapy telangiectatic matting. It has been recommended that the volume injected at each point be limited to 0.5 cc. Minimal injection pressures are also highly recommended. The area of blanching upon injection of the sclerosant at each point should be limited to 1.5 cm.[21]

A retrospective analysis of 2120 patients was performed by Davis and Duffy[23] to determine the risk factors for postsclerotherapy telangiectatic matting. The risk factors identified in more patients with telangiectatic matting included obesity, a history of hormonal therapy during treatment, a history of spider vein development after excess hormonal states, a positive family history, and a longer duration of spider veins.

Telangiectatic matting can be resistant to treatment with sclerotherapy, but the pulsed-dye laser has been used successfully for treatment of post-sclerotherapy telangiectatic matting.[5,20] Since the telangiectatic matting may fade with time, it may be advisable to wait approximately 6 months for the telangiectatic matting to resolve prior to initiating treatment alternatives.

ALLERGIC REACTIONS

True allergic reactions are rare to all the popularly used sclerosants. Vasovagal (syncopal) reactions to the injections themselves are not uncommon, however. One of the advantages to the supine position for the sclerotherapy patient is the elimination of falling when one of these common fainting episodes occurs. These are simply treated by stopping the injections with careful observation of the patient's vital signs and placement of the patient in the Trendelenburg position. It is important to rule out any more serious type of reaction.

True allergic reactions can be characterized as mild, moderate, or severe. These allergic reactions represent immediate-type IgE-mediated hypersensitivity reactions. The serious, life-threatening anaphylactic response occurs within minutes following administration of the antigen and so can be recognized and appropriately treated. The more mild cutaneous manifestations have been noted 8 hours after sclerotherapy.[24] Patients should be warned about the possibility of an allergic reaction so that they can receive the necessary care if it does occur.

Mild symptoms, such as a rash, generalized urticaria (hives), or pruritus can be treated with diphenhydramine (Benadryl) 50 mg PO TID-QID. Benadryl can now be purchased without a prescription. This mild allergic reaction also can be controlled by administration of 0.2 to 0.5 ml of 1:1000 epinephrine subcutaneously, with repeated doses as required at 3-minutes intervals, particularly if one suspects that this may represent only the early signs of a more severe reaction. The generalized urticaria must be differentiated from localized urticaria, which can occur *normally* in the injected area due to the effect of the sclerosant on the endothelium. The generalized pruritic allergic response also must be differentiated from localized itching secondary to the action of the sclerosant, which also occurs quite commonly.[7]

Angioedema, commonly presenting as swelling of the face and tongue, can accompany the urticaria. More moderate reactions can include laryngeal edema, which may present as a "lump in the throat." If stridor is present, diphenhydramine 50 to 80 mg should be given intramuscularly or intravenously in addition to the epinephrine. Bronchospasm presenting as wheezing should be treated additionally with an inhaled bronchodilator or intravenous aminophylline 250 to 500 mg (6 mg/kg) over 10 to 20 minutes. Corticosteroids, such as dexamethasone (Decadron) 8 mg, also should be given intravenously. The corticosteroids are not effective for treatment of the acute episode but may help prevent recurrence of the symptoms later.[25,26] Oxygen via a nasal cannula may be helpful, but endotracheal intubation or tracheostomy may be required if respiratory compromise worsens.

In the most serious type of reaction, the sequence of urticaria, angioedema, and bronchospasm can be followed by cardiovascular collapse secondary to profound systemic vasodilatation. As the reaction progresses, the same protocol is followed as described above. However, if the patient does not respond to these emergency measures but continues to worsen with the development of hypotension, an intravenous line should be started as soon as possible so that the epinephrine can be given intravenously, as well as intravenous fluids. Then 0.5 to 1 ml of epinephrine 1:1000 is diluted to 5-10 ml with saline, yielding 5 to 10 ml of a 1:10,000 dilution to be given intravenously, and this can be repeated every 5 minutes. This is given in addition to the diphenhydramine and dexamethasone and, if needed, the aminophylline intravenously, as outlined previously. The patient should be transferred immediately to the hospital and appropriate consultations obtained for continuing critical care.

These protocols for treating allergic reactions should be readily available where sclerotherapy is being performed (Table 8–1). The office must be equipped with an emergency kit containing all the medications listed, as well as intravenous lines and fluids. One person in the office must be designated to review the stock of emergency medicines periodically so as to replace any outdated medications.

TENDER THROMBI AND THROMBOPHLEBITIS

Larger reticular veins of 3 to 4 mm will more frequently develop larger thrombi that feel nodular to palpation and can be tender.[8] The inci-

TABLE 8–1. *Treatment of Allergic Reactions*

Type of Reaction	Clinical Signs	Treatment
Mild	Rash Hives Itching	Diphenhydramine (Benadryl) 50 mg PO TID-QID OR Epinephrine 1:1,000 0.2–0.5 ml SC (may repeat Q 3min)
Moderate	Swelling of face or tongue or stridor	Epinephrine 1:1,000 0.2–0.5 ml SC (may repeat Q 3-min) Diphenhydramine (Benadryl) 50–80 mg IM or IV
	Wheezing	Aminophylline 250– 500 mg 6 mg/kg) over 10–20 min IV Dexamethason (Decadron) 8 mg IV
Severe	Anaphylactic shock	Epinephrine 5–10 ml of 1:10,000 IV. (0.5–1 ml of Epinephrine 1:1,000 diluted to 5-10 ml with saline). May repeat at 5 min Diphenhydramine (Benadryl) 50 mg IV, Dexamethasone (Decadron) 8 mg IV IV fluids
	Wheezing	Aminophylline 250–500 mg (6 mg/kg) Oxygen nasal cannula or endotracheal intubation or tracheostomy Hospitalization

dence has been reported as 5.375 percent in one series.[27] The most frequent sequela of thrombi is hyperpigmentation. Clot evacuation, as shown in Figure 8–2, usually eliminates the tenderness and minimizes the hyperpigmentation.

Superficial thrombophlebitis has been noted in less than 1 to 5 percent of postsclerotherapy patients and also usually occurs in larger reticular veins.[8,27] This can be treated conservatively with ambulation, aspirin, and warm compresses and usually resolves rapidly within a week.

Because of the higher incidence of thrombi and thrombophlebitis in larger reticular veins, these may be treated alternatively by ambulatory phlebectomy rather than sclerotherapy. In this newer technique, a tiny stab incision is made overlying the reticular vein, which is delivered into this tiny incision using specially designed hooks.[28] Visible segments of vein are avulsed through these multiple tiny stab incisions along the vein path.

DEEP VEIN THROMBOSIS

Deep vein thrombosis after sclerotherapy of spider veins is exceedingly rare, with two cases having been reported.[29–31] Communication between spider veins and deep veins of the legs has been demonstrated by a direct injection of the superficial telangiectasias with radiopaque medium. This was visualized radiographically draining into the deep venous system in 2 of 15 patients in one study.[32] In order to help prevent deep venous thrombosis, it was recommended that the volume of sclerosant per injection site be limited to less than 0.5 cc based on the findings of this study. Even though this complication is rare, it should be discussed with the patient, since it is a potentially fatal complication if pulmonary embolism results.

REFERENCES

1. Goldman MP, Kaplan RP, Duffy DM. Postsclerotherapy hyperpigmentation: A histologic evaluation. J Dermatol Surg Oncol 1987; 13:547–550.
2. Tretbar LL. Injection sclerotherapy for spider telangiectasias: A 20–year experience with sodium tetradecyl sulfate. J Dermatol Surg Oncol 1989; 15: 223–225.
3. Bodian E. Sclerotherapy. Dialogues Dermatol 1983; 13(3):(tape).
4. Alderman DB. Therapy for essential cutaneous telangiectasia. Postgrad Med 1977; 61:91–95.
5. Weiss RA, Weiss MA. Incidence of side effects in the treatment of telangiectasias by compression sclerotherapy: Hypertonic saline vs polidocanol. J Dermatol Surg Oncol 1990; 16:800–804.
6. Cacciatore E. Experience of sclerotherapy with Aethoxysklérol. Minerva Cardioangiol 1979; 27:255–262.
7. Carlin MC, Ratz JL. Treatment of telangiectasia: Comparison of sclerosing agents. J Dermatol Surg Oncol 1987; 13:1181–1184.
8. Goldman PM. Sclerotherapy of superficial venules and telangiectasias of the lower extremities. Dermatol Clin 1987; 5:369–379.

9. Bodian EL. Sclerotherapy. Semin Dermatol 1987; 6:238–248.

10. Orbach EJ. Hazards of sclerotherapy of varicose veins—Their prevention and treatment of complications. Vasa 1979; 8:170–173.

11. Goldman MP, Bennett RG. Treatment of telangiectasia: A review. J Am Acad Dermatol 1987; 17:167–182.

12. Goldman MP, Beaudoing D, Marley W, et al. Compression in the treatment of leg telangiectasia: A preliminary report. J Dermatol Surg Oncol 1990; 16:322–325.

13. Georgiev M. Postsclerotherapy hyperpigmentations: A one-year follow-up. J Dermatol Surg Oncol 1990; 16:608–610.

14. Bodian EL. Sclerotherapy: A personal appraisal. J Dermatol Surg Oncol 1989; 15:156–161.

15. Thibault P, Wlodarczyk J. Postsclerotherapy hyperpigmentation: The role of serum ferritin levels and the effectiveness of treatment with the copper vapor laser. J Dermatol Surg Oncol 1992; 18:47–52.

16. Goldman MP. Postsclerotherapy hyperpigmentation: Treatment with a flash-lamp-excited pulsed dye laser. J Dermatol Surg Oncol 1992; 18:417–422.

17. de Groot WP. Treatment of varicose veins: Modern concepts and methods. J Dermatol Surg Oncol 1989; 15:191–198.

18. Goldman MP, Kaplan RP, Oki LN, et al. Extravascular effects of sclerosants in rabbit skin: A clinical and histological examination. J Dermatol Surg Oncol 1986; 12:1085–1088.

19. Hofer AE. Aethoxysklerol (Kreussler) in the sclerosing treatment of varices. Minerva Cardioangiol 1972; 20:601–604.

20. Goldman MP, Fitzpatrick RE. Pulsed-dye laser treatment of leg telangiectasia: With and without simultaneous sclerotherapy. J Dermatol Surg Oncol 1990; 16:338–344.

21. Ouvry PA. Telangiectasia and sclerotherapy. J Dermatol Surg Oncol 1989; 15:177–181.

22. Goldman MP. Compression in the treatment of leg telangiectasia: Theoretical considerations. J Dermatol Surg Oncol 1989; 15:184–188.

23. Davis LT, Duffy DM. Determination of incidence and risk factors for postsclerotherapy telangiectatic matting of the lower extremity: A retrospective analysis. J Dermatol Surg Oncol 1990; 16:327–330.

24. Fronek H, Fronek A, Saltzberg G. Allergic reactions to sotradecol. J Dermatol Surg Oncol 1989; 15:684.

25. Austen KF. Diseases of immediate type hypersensitivity. In Wilson JD, et al, eds: Harrison's Principles of Internal Medicine, 12th ed. New York: McGraw-Hill, 1991, pp 1422–1428.

26. Courtiss EH, Kanter MA. The prevention and management of medical problems during office surgery. Plast Reconstr Surg 1990; 85:127–136.

27. Sadick NS. Treatment of varicose and telangiectatic leg veins with hypertonic saline: A comparative study of heparin and saline. J Dermatol Surg Oncol 1990; 16:24–28.

28. Dortu J, Raymond-Martimbeau P. Ambulatory Phlebectomy. Houston: PRM Editions, 1993, pp 83–98.

29. Beresford SAA, Chant ADB, Jones HO, et al. Varicose veins: A comparison of surgery and injection/compression sclerotherapy. Lancet 1978; 1:921–924.

30. Goor W, Leu HJ, Mahler F. Thrombosen in tiéfen venen und in arterian mach varizensklerosierung. Vasa 1987; 16:124–129.

31. Reid RG, Rothnie NG. Treatment of varicose veins by compression sclerotherapy. Br J Surg 1968; 55:889–895.

32. Böhler-Sommeregger K, Karnel F, Schuller-Petrovič S, Santler R. Do telangiectasias communicate with the deep venous system? J Dermatol Surg Oncol 1992; 18:403–406.

ADDITIONAL READINGS

Atlas LN. Hazards connected with the treatment of varicose veins. Surg Gynecol Obstet 1943; 77:136–140.

Chatard H. Pigmentations post-sclérothérapiques. Phlébologie 1976; 29: 211–216.

Cuttell PJ, Fox JA. The aetiology and treatment of varicose pigmentation. Phlebologie 1982; 35:381–389.

Fegan WG. The complications of compression sclerotherapy. Practitioner 1971; 207:797–799.

Feuerstein W. Anaphylactic reaction to hydroxypolyaethoxydodecon. Vasa 1973; 2:292–294.

Goldstein M. Les complications de la sclerotherapie. Phlébologie 1979; 32:221–228.

MacGowan WAL. Sclerotherapy-Prevention of accidents: A review. J R Soc Med 1985; 78:136–137.

Orbach EJ. The importance of removal of postinjection coagula during the course of sclerotherapy of varicose veins. Vasa 1974; 3:475–477.

Puissegur-Lupo ML. Sclerotherapy: Review of results and complications in 200 patients. J Dermatol Surg Oncol 1989; 15:214–219.

Sigg K. The treatment of varicosities and accompanying complications. Angiology 1952; 3:355–379.

Wallois P. Incidents et accidents au cours du traitment sclerosant des varices et leur prevention. Phlebologie 1971; 24:217–224.

Williams RA, Wilson SE. Sclerosant treatment of varicose veins and deep vein thrombosis. Arch Surg 1984; 119:1283–1285.

Zimmet SE. The prevention of cutaneous necrosis following extravasation of hypertonic saline and sodium tetradecyl sulfate. J Dermatol Surg Oncol 1993; 19:641–646.

ALTERNATIVE METHODS OF TREATMENT OF SPIDER VEINS

9

SPIDER VEINS OF THE LEGS differ in etiology and histology from spider telangiectasias commonly found in other areas. The red spider telangiectasias commonly located on the face, neck, and thorax consist chiefly of a central arteriole from which superficial vessels radiate.[1] On the contrary, spider veins of the legs were examined by de Faria and Moraes[2] and found to represent ectatic veins subject to hydrostatic venous pressure.

Three alternative methods to sclerotherapy have been employed for treating telangiectasias in all areas of the body: (1) dermabrasion, (2) electrosurgery, and (3) laser therapy. These three modalities have been successful in treating arteriolar-type spider telangiectasias such as occur on the face and upper body. Of these three modalities, however, only laser therapy has shown some potential for treating spider veins of the lower extremities. The differences in the success rates of these three modalities in treating telangiectasias of the face and upper body versus spider veins of the legs may be related to the difference in etiology, histology, and pathology of these two different conditions. These modalities may not achieve adequate vessel obliteration, leading to reopening of vessel lumina when subjected to the hydrostatic venous pressure in the legs, accounting for poor results and high recurrence rates when treating spider veins of the legs. Complications of these modalities also have been more significant in the legs than in other areas. These factors all account for the failure of other methods of treating telangiectasias elsewhere to replace sclerotherapy as the preferred method of treatment of spider veins of the legs.

DERMABRASION

Dermabrasion has been reported to be effective for treating telangiectasias on the nose related to x-ray and actinic damage.[3] Although dermabrasion is a well-recognized technique for the treatment of actinic keratoses, it has not been widely accepted for treatment of telangiectasias alone. Because of the potential for scarring and pigment changes in the legs, it is not a recommended treatment for spider veins of the legs.

ELECTROSURGERY

Punctate electrocautery of the central arterioles of spider telangiectasias of the face and upper body has been used widely for obliteration of these lesions.[4,5] Electrosurgery results in ablation of the telangiectasias mechanically, either by dehydration (electrodesiccation) or heat (electrocautery). The electrosurgical needle is placed through the skin into the telangiectasia, and the switch is lightly tripped for a second at a very low amperage. In order to avoid injury to the skin surface, Kobayashi[6] in Japan developed partially insulated needles that protect the skin surface from damage by insulation at the proximal end. Partially insulated microneedles are available for electrocautery units in the United States from Elmed, Inc. Because electrosurgery acts on such a very localized area, the scarring and pigmentary changes that would result make it impractical for treatment of spider veins of the lower extremities.

LASER THERAPY

The treatment of vascular skin lesions by laser has been in a state of evolution since it was first introduced in the 1960s. *Laser* is an acronym

Simplified Medical Laser

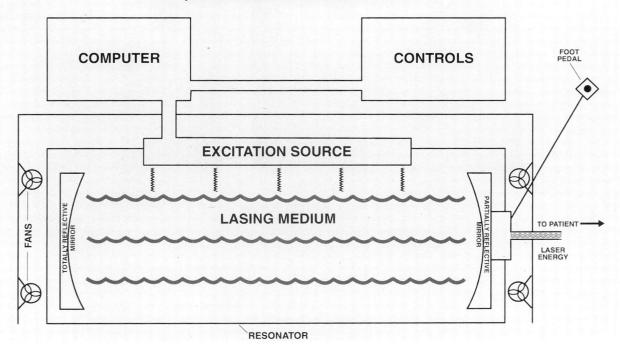

FIGURE 9–1.
Diagram of medical laser.
(Courtesy of K. Anderson)

for light amplification by stimulated emission of radiation. All lasers operate according to a similar principle. An excitation source stimulates the emission of photons in the laser medium. This generates the laser beam, which consists of light of a single wavelength (monochromatic) traveling in coherent (synchronous), collimated (nondivergent) waves (Fig. 9–1). The color of the laser light depends on the wavelength. Certain pigments will preferentially absorb light of certain wavelengths, resulting in the release of radiant energy, causing thermal destruction. For example, the blue-green light emitted by the argon laser is absorbed by the red pigment of oxyhemoglobin. The light emitted by other lasers, such as the CO_2 and Yag, is absorbed ubiquitously by water resulting in nonspecific tissue destruction.

Because of this nonspecificity of the CO_2 laser, the results of its use in treating spider veins of the legs were disappointing. The response was inferior to sclerotherapy, coupled with hypopigmented scarring and a high recurrence rate. In addition, patients preferred sclerotherapy.[7,8]

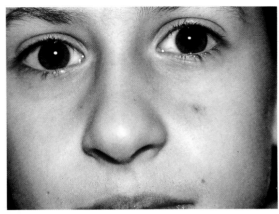
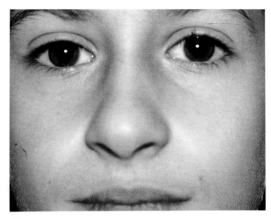

A   B

FIGURE 9–2. *A. Typical spider telangiectasia of the cheek. B. Seven months after successful eradication of spider telangiectasia of the cheek with the flashlamp pulsed dye laser in one treatment. (Courtesy of Dr. A. Reilly).*

Even the argon laser, with some specificity for oxyhemoglobin, showed poor response in treatment of spider veins of the legs.[9]

The blue-green argon laser light also has significant melanin absorption at 488 and 514 nm. More recently, the yellow-light lasers (575 to 595 nm wavelength) were felt to be superior for the treatment of cutaneous vascular disorders. The yellow light penetrates to the depth of the dermal blood vessels, so it is more specifically absorbed by hemoglobin with less melanin absorption.[10,11] These yellow-light lasers include the flashlamp pulsed dye laser (Candela), the copper vapor laser, and argon pumped tunable dye laser. These lasers are extremely effective for eradicating spider telangiectasias on the face (Fig. 9–2). The pulsed dye laser also has been used successfully to treat fine-caliber red telangiectasias (less than 0. 2 mm in diameter) on the legs, including postsclerotherapy telangiectatic matting.[12] It was postulated in this study that the satisfactory results may have been influenced by the strict selection criteria; that is, the patients who responded well had only fine-caliber red telangiectasias with no associated feeding reticular veins.

As laser technology progresses, selective vascular destruction without thermal injury to the surrounding tissue may become possible, perhaps through the use of new cooling devices recently developed for use with lasers.[13] Notwithstanding the results of therapy, the purpura that

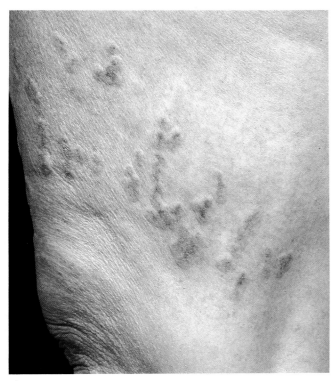

A

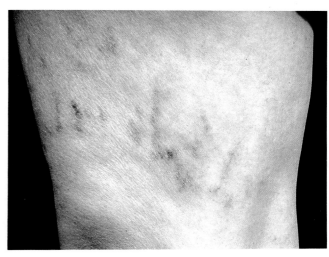

B

FIGURE 9–3. *A. Typical appearance of thighs 1 week after treatment of fine spider veins with the flashlamp pulsed dye laser. B. Typical appearance 3 weeks after treatment with laser. The posttreatment reaction is usually more noticeable and longer-lasting after laser treatment of spider veins of the legs than after sclerotherapy.*

develops following laser therapy is much more noticeable and takes much longer to fade than the mild initial bruising after sclerotherapy (Fig. 9–3). For now, sclerotherapy remains the most widely accepted method for obliteration of spider veins of the legs.

REFERENCES

1. Bean WB. Vascular Spiders and Related Lesions of the Skin. Springfield, IL: Charles C Thomas, 1958.
2. de Faria JL, Moraes IN. Histopathology of the telangiectasia associated with varicose veins. Dermatologica 1963; 127:321–329.
3. Lapins NA. Dermabrasion for telangiectasia. J Dermatol Surg Oncol 1983; 9:470–472.

4. Mulliken JB. Capillary and other telangiectatic stains. In Mulliken JB, Young AE. Vascular Birthmarks: Hemangiomas and Malformations. Philadelphia: WB Saunders, 1988, pp 170–195.

5. Burdick K. Electrocautery of minor skin lesions. In Epstein E, Epstein E Jr, eds: Skin Surgery, 5th ed. Springfield, IL: Charles C Thomas, 1982, pp 419–426.

6. Kobayashi T. Electrosurgery using insulated needles: Treatment of telangiectasias. J Dermatol Surg Oncol 1986; 12:936–942.

7. Apfelberg DB, Maser MR, Lash H., et al. Use of the argon and carbon dioxide lasers for treatment of superficial venous varicosities of the lower extremity. Lasers Surg Med 1984; 4:221–232.

8. Pfeifer JR, Hawtof GD. Injection sclerotherapy and CO_2 laser sclerotherapy in the ablation of cutaneous spider veins of the lower extremity. Phlebology 1989; 4:231–240.

9. Craig RDP, Purser JM, Lessells AM, et al. Argon laser therapy for cutaneous lesions. Br J Plast Surg 1985; 38:148–155.

10. McDaniel D. Cutaneous vascular disorders: Advances in laser treatment. Cutis 1990; 45:339–360.

11. Polla LL, Tan OT, Garden JM, et al. Tunable pulsed-dye laser for the treatment of benign cutaneous vascular ectasia. Dermatologica 1987; 174:11–17.

12. Goldman MP, Fitzpatrick RE. Pulsed-dye laser treatment of leg telangiectasia: With and without simultaneous sclerotherapy. J Dermatol Surg Oncol 1990; 16:338–344.

13. Chess C, Chess Q. Cool laser optics treatment of large telangiectasia of the lower extremities. J Dermatol Surg Oncol 1993; 19:74–80.

ADDITIONAL READINGS

Anderson RR, Jaenicke KF, Parrish JA. Mechanisms of selective vascular changes caused by dye lasers. Lasers Surg Med 1983; 3:211–215.

Apfelberg DB, Smith T, Maser MR, et al. Study of three laser systems for treatment of superficial varicosities of the lower extremity. Lasers Surg Med 1987; 7:219–223.

Bonafé JL, Laffitte F, Chavoin JP, et al. Hyperpigmentation induced by argon laser therapy of hemangiomas: Optical and electron microscopic studies. Dermatologica 1985; 170:225–229.

Garden JM, Tan OT, Polla L, et al. The pulse-dye laser as a modality for treating cutaneous small blood vessel disease processes. Lasers Surg Med 1986; 6:259–260.

Greenwald J, Rosen S, Anderson RR, et al. Comparative histological studies of the tunable dye (at 577 nm) laser and argon laser: The specific vascular effects of the dye laser. J Invest Dermatol 1981; 77:305–310.

Kaplan I, Peled I. The carbon dioxide laser in the treatment of superficial telangiectasias. Br J Plast Surg 1975; 28:214–215.

Kirsch N. Telangiectasia and electrolysis (letter). J Dermatol Surg Oncol 1984; 10:9–10.

Lanthaler M, Haina D, Waidelich W, Braun-Falco O. Laser therapy of venous lakes (Bean-Walsh) and telangiectasias. Plast Reconstr Surg 1984; 73:78–83.

Lyons GD, Owens RE, Mouney DF. Argon laser destruction of cutaneous telangiectatic lesions. Laryngoscope 1981; 91:1322–1325.

Ratz JL, Goldman L, Bauman WE. Posttreatment complications of the argon laser. Arch Dermatol 1985; 121:714.

Recoules-Arché J. Electrocoagulation. Phlebologie 1966; 33:885–892.

Tan OT, Carney JM, Margolis R, et al. Histologic responses of port-wine stains treated by argon, carbon dioxide, and tunable dye lasers: A preliminary report. Arch Dermatol 1986; 122:1016–1022.

Waner M, Dinehart SM, Wilson MB, et al. A comparison of copper vapor and flashlamp-pumped dye lasers in the treatment of facial telangiectasia. J Dermatol Surg Oncol 1993; 19:992–998.

OTHER AESTHETIC SCLEROTHERAPY APPLICATIONS

10

TELANGIECTASIAS OCCUR frequently on the face, particularly in the perialar areas and on the cheeks. At times, these can represent a cutaneous manifestation of a systemic disease or can overlie a basal cell carcinoma; however, in the large majority of cases, their occurrence is idiopathic. Various modalities for treating facial telangiectasias, including electrocauterization and laser therapy, have yielded consistently favorable results.[1–3] Consequently, the need for sclerotherapy as another modality for treatment of facial telangiectasias is uncommon.

Ulcerations on the face have been described as a result of sclerotherapy.[4] The resulting scars, although small, are much less tolerated on the face than they are on the legs. Consequently, sclerotherapy is used with reservation on the face. It is used primarily to ablate extensive "blue" telangiectasias on the face suggestive of a venous origin. Although various sclerosing agents have been described for use on the face, I prefer weak concentrations of polidocanol because of its minimal risk of ulceration.[4,5] Dramatic results can be achieved safely with the use of 0.25% to 0.5% polidocanol for sclerotherapy of facial spider veins (Fig. 10–1).

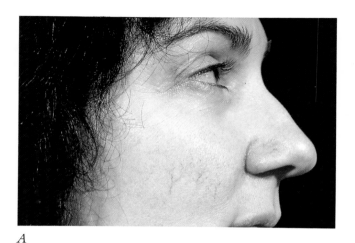

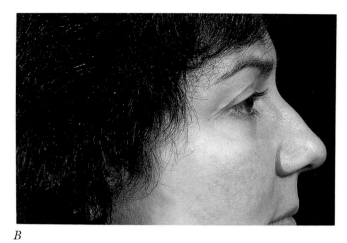

A   B

FIGURE 10–1. *A. Before sclerotherapy. B. Two months after sclerotherapy with 0.25% polidocanol in two treatment sessions. (Courtesy of Dr. P. Schneider.)*

Telangiectasias can result following trauma or undermining of the skin, such as after rhinoplasty or following tissue expansion. Sclerotherapy is, again, one of several treatment options, including laser and electrocauterization. Sclerotherapy has the advantages of its ease and minimal expense and equipment required compared to the alternative methods of treatment. It is limited by the size of the telangiectasias that can be entered with a 30–gauge needle; however, with practice, one can inject intravascularly telangiectasias that appear to be smaller than the 30–gauge needle itself. Figure 10–2 shows one example of spider veins of the arm that developed following tissue expansion. In this case, tissue-expanded skin was used to replace a large skin-grafted area on the arm and forearm following a severe avulsion injury. Subsequently, sclerotherapy with 0.5% polidocanol successfully obliterated these spider veins on the expanded flaps in two sessions 4 weeks apart.

Sclerotherapy also has been used in the treatment of hemangiomas, venous malformations, and multiple glomangiomas.[6–8] All these vascular malformations can be very disfiguring because of the large bulk, gross discoloration, and involvement of large areas. Their large size and extensive area involvement make surgical resection impossible without extensive scarring or sacrifice of important structures. More conservative treatment is preferable to debulk these disfiguring malformations.

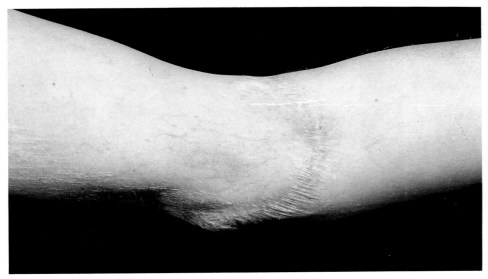

A

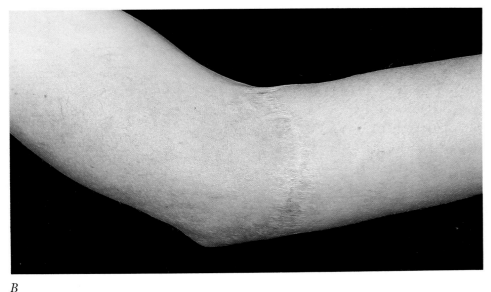

B

FIGURE 10–2.
A. Spider veins of arm that developed following tissue expansion for coverage of a previously skin-grafted area. B. Six months after sclerotherapy with 0.5% polidocanol in two treatment sessions.

Various treatment modalities have included selective embolization combined with surgery, systemic or intralesional treatment with steroids, and intralesional sclerotherapy.[9,10] Figure 10–3 shows a case of multiple glomangiomas of the upper extremity that appear clinically as multiple nodular blue tumors and add great bulk to the upper extremity by their sheer number. Each of these vascular spaces was injected with 0.1 to 0.2 cc of 0.25% polidocanol. In many cases, a blood return could be obtained prior to injection. The treatment sessions at first

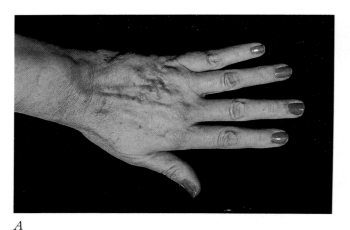

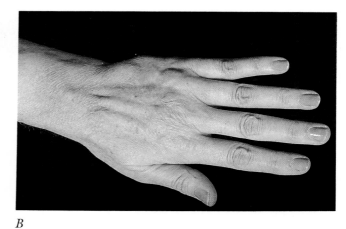

A

B

FIGURE 10–3.
A. Multiple glomangiomas of the hand. B. One year after sclerotherapy with 0.25% polidocanol in five treatment sessions.

were limited to regional areas because of the large number of lesions that involved the entire upper extremity. Four weeks were allowed before repeating sclerotherapy in any one area, and each area was injected five times over 5 months. A dramatic improvement in tumor bulk was obtained (Fig. 10–3).

The conditions discussed in this chapter occur less frequently than spider veins of the lower extremities. Nonetheless, in these cases, sclerotherapy can also result in a significant aesthetic improvement with little cost, effort, or risk of complications.

REFERENCES

1. Mulliken JB. Capillary and other telangiectatic stains. In Mulliken JB, Young AE. Vascular Birthmarks: Hemangiomas and Malformations. Philadelphia: WB Saunders, 1988, pp 170–195.

2. Burdick K. Electrocautery of minor skin lesions. In Epstein E, Epstein E Jr, eds: Skin Surgery, 5th ed. Springfield, IL: Charles C Thomas, 1982, pp 419–426.

3. Ruiz-Esparza J, Goldman MP, Fitzpatrick RE, et al. Flash lamp-pumped dye laser treatment of telangiectasia. J Dermatol Surg Oncol 1993; 19:1000–1003.

4. Bodian EL. Sclerotherapy: A personal appraisal. J Dermatol Surg Oncol 1989; 15:156–161.

5. Hofer AE. Aethoxysklérol (Kreussler) in the sclerosing treatment of varices. Minerva Cardioangiol 1972; 20:601–604.

6. Woods JE. Extended use of sodium tetradecyl sulfate in treatment of hemangiomas and other related conditions. Plast Reconstr Surg 1987; 79:542–549.

7. Govrin-Yehudain J, Moscona AR, Calderon N, Hirshowitz B. Treatment of hemangiomas by sclerosing agents: An experimental and clinical study. Ann Plast Surg 1987; 18:465–469.

8. Gould EP. Sclerotherapy for multiple glomangiomata. J Dermatol Surg Oncol 1991; 17:351–352.

9. Leikensohn JR, Epstin LI, Vasconez LO. Superselective embolization and surgery of noninvoluting hemangiomas and A-V malformations. Plast Reconstr Surg 1981; 68:143–152.

10. Brown SH, Neerhout RC, Fonkalsrud EW. Prednisone therapy in the management of large hemangiomas in infants and children. Surgery 1972; 71:168–173.

ADDITIONAL READINGS

Lewis JR. The treatment of hemangiomas. Plast Reconstr Surg 1957;19:201–212.

Minkow B, Laufer D, Gutman P. Treatment of oral hemangiomas with local sclerosing agents. Int J Oral Surg 1979; 8:18–21.

Stockdale CR. Peripheral angiomas and their treatment with sclerosing solution. Oral Surg 1959; 12:1157–1162.

INDEX